The Spasmodic Torticollis Handbook

A Guide to Treatment and Rehabilitation

MAYANK PATHAK, MD
KAREN FREI, MD
DANIEL TRUONG, MD

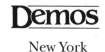

New York

Demos Medical Publishing, 386 Park Avenue South, New York, New York 10016

Library of Congress Cataloging-in-Publication Data

Pathak, Mayank.
  Spasmodic torticollis handbook : a guide to treatment and rehabilitation / Mayank Pathak, Karen Frei, Daniel Truong.
      p. ; cm.
Includes index.
  ISBN 1-888799-77-3 (pbk.)
  1. Torticollis–Popular works.
  [DNLM: 1. Torticollis–Popular Works. WE 708 P297s 2003] I. Frei, Karen. II. Truong, Daniel, M.D. III. Title.
  RC935.D8P38 2003
  617.5'3–dc21

                                                                      2003000151

Printed in the United States of America.

Visit the Demos Medical Publishing web site at www.demosmedpub.com

Contents

Preface

Spasmodic torticollis, also known as cervical dystonia, is a relatively rare neurologic disorder that is not as familiar to the general population as are more common movement disorders such as Parkinson's Disease. Indeed, it is only vaguely recognized by most physicians not specializing in neurology; as a result, many of our patients had their disorder for years before a definitive diagnosis was made. Spasmodic torticollis affects about three people in 10,000, or an estimated 85,000 individuals in the United States alone. Despite this, there has been a lack of information sources outside of the professional medical literature for use by affected individuals and their families. It is for this reason that we undertook the development of this book

Because of the difficulty in referring our patients to outside sources of information, we began working with the National Spasmodic Torticollis Association (NSTA) to develop educational and reference materials appropriate for laypersons. This book is designed to provide comprehensive information on the disorder for people with spasmodic torticollis and those close to them. Medical terms and concepts are introduced sequentially and then used as building blocks for the later discussion. Thus, although we have provided an extensive glossary, we suggest that you read each of the chapters in order.

Our intent is to first present a clear definition of the disorder, categorize it appropriately as a movement disorder that is part of the broader category of neurologic diseases, and to differentiate it from other conditions with which it is often confused. We then present a stepwise introduction to the relevant anatomy and physiology of the nervous system and neck. We have drawn on the stories of scores of our patients to build a progressive depiction of the experiences an individual might have as he or she goes through the initial onset of symptoms, progression of the disorder, seeking medical care, diagnosis, treatment, and subsequent outcome. Personal vignettes from the experiences of selected patients are provided where they illustrate particular points in the discussion.

Subsequent chapters discuss various modes of treatment for spasmodic torticollis. Prior to the mid- 1980's, there were no specific treatments for this disorder. Nearly all treatment consisted of using oral medications that were primarily intended for other medical conditions. Since most of these medications are still in use, and a few new ones have been added, a chapter is devoted to detailing them and discussing the general principles of medication therapy. During the past decade, a more specific intervention, chemodenervation using botulinum toxin, has become the primary and most effective treatment for spasmodic torticollis. More familiar to the public as a cosmetic treatment for wrinkles, there is little awareness of botulinum toxin as a treatment for movement disorders. We have redressed this problem in the treatment section of this book. Additionally, for those few patients requiring surgery, we provide a description of neurosurgical techniques developed during the last twenty years specifically for the treatment of spasmodic torticollis.

The final chapter of this book is a manual of therapeutic rehabilitation exercises. Our patients repeatedly ask us if any exercises or rehabilitative techniques can alleviate their symptoms. Although spasmodic torticollis is discussed in texts used by physical therapists, and there are books of exercises for general neck pain, until now there has been no patient-oriented manual of exercises specifically designed to alleviate the symptoms of torticollis. For these reasons, we developed a group of exercises that can be performed by most patients without assistance and using a bare minimum of equipment.

We first presented these exercises in a videotape, *Physical Therapy and Exercises for Spasmodic Torticollis.* In this book, we present these exercises in the same order and format used in the videotape. This book may thus be used alone to learn the exercises, or used in conjunction with the videotape. Since each person's case of spasmodic torticollis is different, only certain of the exercises are appropriate for them. We advise you to read through each of the exercises in the chapter. Each contains a description of the particular muscles and type of abnormal neck position that it is intended to treat. You can thus identify which exercises are appropriate for you. You should discuss the exercises with your physical therapist if you have one.

Please obtain permission from your doctor before beginning any of the exercises.

The figures in this book were drawn by Dr. Pathak, who has strived to accurately represent subtle differences in head and neck position without making the drawings either too complex or too simple. Examine closely the neck and shoulders in the drawings, as particular muscles relevant to each posture or movement have been emphasized.

M. Pathak, MD
K. Frei, MD
D. Truong, MD

Acknowledgments

None of the authors has personally suffered with spasmodic torti-collis; we thus acknowledge and give profuse thanks to our patient Nancy Muller, whose personal account of her illness, given its own chapter herein, has lent this book a personal touch from a first-hand perspective. We also acknowledge and thank those of our patients who gave us their personal experiences to use as vignettes, and all of those and their loved ones from whom we have gleaned knowledge over the years. We thank our colleague, Dr. Steve Jenkins, for review-ing and assisting with the manuscript, Diane Truong for administra-tive support, and Bharti Pathak for logistical assistance.

1

What Is Spasmodic Torticollis?

BASICS

You are reading this book presumably because you suffer from tremor, abnormal unwanted movements, or crooked posture of your head and neck. This is an uncommon condition, and you may have been suspected of having a number of underlying causes for it. A number of different medical conditions may manifest as an abnormal head and neck posture, and the term *torticollis* is loosely applied to many of them. In fact, torticollis simply means "twisted neck." This book deals specifically with the neurologic condition known as *spasmodic torticollis* (ST), also known as *cervical dystonia*. Other causes of abnormal posture will be briefly discussed to differentiate them from ST.

Gathering information is the first step in managing any chronic disorder. By reading this book, you will learn about factors that may cause this condition, how this condition manifests itself, how it progresses, and medications that are used to treat it, as well as exercises that may help you to maintain flexibility and control the pain that may accompany ST. Also included are some tips from other people suffering from ST. This book will serve as a reference for you to share with your doctor and family.

For purposes of the discussion in this book, we provide the following definition: Spasmodic torticollis is a neurologic disorder that results in an involuntary turning or twisting of the head and neck, causing them to assume a forced abnormal posture. It is difficult for the person with ST to voluntarily move his or her head back to a normal straight position. In order to give you a thorough understanding of your disorder, we will first examine the above definition in detail and establish a basic vocabulary.

Neurologic disorders are those that affect the nervous system: the brain, the spinal cord, and the nerves that extend out of the spinal cord to the rest of the body (Figure 1). *Sensory nerves* are those that bring sensory information from the body to the spinal cord to be relayed to the brain (a few sensory nerves, such as those from the ears and eyes, deliver information directly to the brain). *Motor nerves* are those that send information from the brain directly or via the spinal cord to muscles of the body. It is through the motor nerves that muscles are made to contract and cause movement in a particular body part. In general, the brain and spinal cord are referred to as the *central nervous system* (CNS); the motor and sensory nerves are referred to as the *peripheral nervous system.*

The brain contains a number of different types of cells. Those that receive, relay, or send information in the form of electrical and chemical signals are called *neurons.* Certain areas of the brain contain groups of neurons whose main activity is to send, control, or

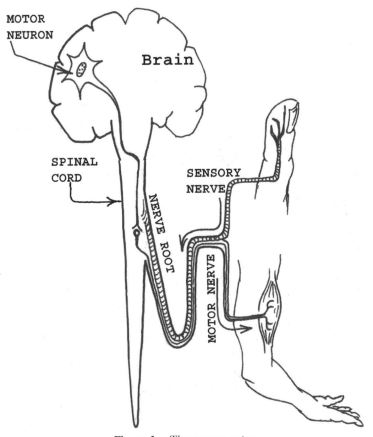

Figure 1   *The nervous system.*

modify information that is sent out through the motor nerves to the muscles. These brain areas, their neurons, and their signal pathways through the spinal cord and motor nerves to the muscles are collectively known as the *motor system.*

Neurologic disorders that affect mainly the motor system are known as *movement disorders.* Movement disorders affect the body's movement and can result in increased stiffness of a limb or other body part due to an increase in the normal resting tone of muscles (rigidity), a slowing down of the normal speed of movements, or an incoordination or loss of dexterity in movements. Some movement disorders may involve an excess of unwanted or difficult-to-control movements, such as tremors or abnormal contorted postures in affected body parts. *Parkinson's disease* is one of the most well known movement disorders. Its symptoms include a slowing down of movements, tremors, and rigidity. Movement disorders that involve mainly an increase in muscle tone and that cause sustained abnormal postures in affected body parts are called *dystonias.* If the affected body part also has tremor, writhing movements, or other uncontrollable motion, the disorder may also be called a *dyskinesia.*

ST is thus a dystonia that mainly affects the muscles of the neck. It may also be termed a dyskinesia if there is abnormal neck motion. The word "spasmodic" indicates abnormal contractions, or spasms, of various muscles that bring about the contorted position. The primary abnormality in ST is not in the neck, however. It is currently believed that the underlying problem is in the motor system of the CNS, specifically in a part of the motor system called the *basal ganglia.* Abnormal signals from the brain cause the head and neck to assume an involuntary contorted posture. The word *involuntary* should be stressed here. This means that the affected individual is not voluntarily, or volitionally, moving his or her head into the abnormal posture. He or she may have to exert voluntary effort to try to bring the head back to normal position, but when that effort is stopped, his or her head will return to the abnormal position. The neck is also known by its Latin name, cervix, and thus another term for ST is *cervical dystonia.*

THE SYMPTOMS AND CLINICAL COURSE

Now that you have an understanding of the definition of ST, we will go over the signs and symptoms of this disorder in more detail.

ST may begin at any age, but appears most often between the ages 25 to 55 years. It affects men and women about equally, and has no predilection for any particular race or ethnic group. The disorder usually develops gradually. Neck discomfort, mild pain, and a feeling of stiffness may be the earliest symptoms. Muscle contractions may produce subtle jerking movements of the head that resemble a tremor. These early manifestations may not be present all of the time. They may occur only when the individual is fatigued, such as at the end of the day; or may appear transiently during or after physical stress or exercise; or during anxiety or emotional stress. There may be a subtle tilt to the head, but individuals at this stage are seldom aware of their torticollis as a distinct medical disorder. They usually believe they are experiencing "muscle tension," and treat themselves with over-the-counter pain medications, massage, rest, and sometimes chiropractic care.

When the symptoms persist, they may see their primary physician. Unless the signs of the disorder are obvious at this point, they may then, appropriately, receive conservative treatments with prescription pain medications, muscle relaxants, and possibly referral to a physical therapist or chiropractor. Sometimes, in mild cases, these conservative measures may be all that are required to keep the symptoms at a reasonably tolerable level, even if a definitive diagnosis of ST has not been made. In many cases, however, the disorder progresses over months, or even a few years. The symptoms become more continuous and persistent. Head and neck position becomes more contorted and the abnormal posture is obvious to the patient and to others. Pain and stiffness may increase, and pain medications or muscle relaxants may no longer be affective. It becomes increasingly difficult to voluntarily move the head back to neutral position. Head tremor may increase, resembling a nodding "yes-yes" or a shaking "no-no" motion. Occasionally, the dystonia can spread to adjacent body parts such as the shoulders, arms, hands, or the back and spine. In very rare cases, severe dystonia can affect the entire body.

Depending on the severity that the disorder eventually reaches, the twisted posture and pain begin to interfere with a person's normal functioning. An affected person might have trouble shaving, combing his or her hair, or applying makeup, especially if there is significant tremor. It may become more difficult to read, watch television, or drive. Job performance may be impaired. Social interactions may also suffer. This may be due to the individual's own self-conscious embarrassment. It can also be due to aversion or avoidance by strangers, coworkers, or acquaintances; the individual may be assumed by others to have a psychiatric disorder.

Occasionally, especially early in the course of the disease, symptoms of ST will spontaneously remit. In a few cases, remission may be complete and permanent. In the majority of cases, however, the symptoms will reappear at a later date, and the ST becomes a chronic permanent disorder. The general observation has been made that the greater the length of time that symptoms have been present, the more likely that the condition will be permanent. The ST almost never resolves if symptoms have been present for more than one or two years. Its slow progression usually reaches a plateau after about five years, at which point symptoms become stable.

In the chronic stage, the severity of symptoms varies from day to day. Symptoms tend to worsen with fatigue, heavy exercise, and stress, while sleep and relaxation tend to reduce them. Many people find relief by lying on their back, although this is not true for everyone. The neck movements always stop during sleep and, for some people, they do not reappear for a period of time after awakening. This is referred to as the "honeymoon period," and can last from a few minutes to a few hours. The length of the honeymoon period tends to shrink as time goes by. Neck pain may become the predominant symptom.

■

CASE 1

Sam first began to notice head shaking when he was 40 years of age. In fact, his family first noticed he was shaking his head as if in disagreement several months before he realized something was wrong. They noticed that his head shook off and on, especially when he was driving. His coworkers also noticed this and wondered why he shook his head "no" so often. Sam did not realize his head was shaking until one day he noticed he was looking to the right all the time. It became more difficult to watch television unless his head was supported on the back of his favorite recliner. He wasn't able to read the paper at the breakfast table and had to retreat back to his recliner to do so. He began to have difficulty driving and tended to rest his head on the headrest in order to look straight ahead. He went to his family doctor, who told Sam that he did not know what was wrong and prescribed a course of physical therapy. Sam completed the physical therapy despite feeling worse after the more rigorous exercise, and was no better. Although the head turning was uncomfortable and caused him problems, he decided that there wasn't anything else to do for this condition and resolved to continue the exercises and live with it. Gradually, his neck returned to the neutral position and he remained symptom free for the next 20 years. Then, while he was walking for exercise, Sam noticed his head again pulling to the right. This time, his family doctor sent him to a neurologist specializing in movement disorders, who diagnosed Sam as having ST.

Geste Antagoniste: The "Sensory Trick"

Many people with ST develop a tendency to place their hand on the side of their neck or place their fingers against their chin or cheek. For some reason, a light sensory stimulus on the skin of the head or neck dampens the tremors and reduces the severity of the twisting, making it easier to volitionally hold the head in a neutral position. This is known as a "sensory trick" or *geste antagoniste*. Most patients discover this for themselves without needing to be taught. They tend to use this method when reading, watching television, or eating. Unfortunately, the effect of the geste antagoniste is temporary, and full symptoms return as soon as the stimulus is removed. The sensory trick has different levels of effect for different individuals, and not everyone can benefit from it. The exact location of the area to be used and the way in which it is pressed or touched also differs. Some people find relief by putting a hand on the back of their neck. This may also be considered a geste antagoniste, although its mechanism of benefit may be different, having more to do with supporting the head; they may also find relief by lying down on their back. If you have not yet found an effective sensory trick, it may take some experimentation to find one that is effective for you.

Social Embarrassment

ST is a very noticeable medical disorder. When we think of those chronic neurologic illnesses that are perceived by our patients as creating a social stigma, few are as immediately obvious to casual observers as ST. Epilepsy shows no outward signs unless the patient has an attack while being observed. Even Parkinson's disease may not be noticeable in its early stages, until tremor becomes more pronounced. Even then, Parkinson's disease has only a mild to moderate effect on the face, head, and neck. Among neurologic disorders, only paraplegia, with the patient using a wheelchair, is as obvious to all observers. However, paraplegia is rarely perceived as having a psychiatric component, and it is recognizable to most laypersons as the result (usually) of some physical injury. Wheelchair users are more familiar to laypeople, especially given the extensive media coverage of celebrity spinal cord injury during the 1990s. Parkinson's disease also has received public attention of late. Due to this awareness and the current age of "political correctness," strangers tend to be, or at least appear to be, fairly at ease around persons with these disorders.

The situation is not so easy for people with ST, whose disorder remains rare and obscure. Our face, head, and neck are the most visible parts of our bodies, and it is with these that we do most of our communicating. Not only our verbal output, but also our facial expressions and head movements, are continuously used—overtly and subtly—to interact with other people. Spasmodic torticollis disrupts this communication in a very obvious way, especially if the dystonia also involves facial muscles. It is impossible to hide. Add to this the fact that people with ST are often perceived as having an underlying psychiatric condition, and you can see that this disorder can severely impair social interactions.

Our patients who are diagnosed with ST share many of the responses of patients diagnosed with any chronic disease. They wonder how the disorder will affect their employment or professional lives, and how it will affect their personal and sexual relationships. Self-consciousness and social embarrassment can cause patients to become socially disengaged, give up public activities, and may become as disabling as the physical symptoms of the disease. Social embarrassment is one of the "hidden symptoms" of ST. Some patients become clinically depressed, although this condition is not as common with ST as with Parkinson's disease or stroke.

In our years of treating patients with disabling neurologic conditions, including paraplegia, Parkinson's disease, and stroke, we have seen these common initial reactions to becoming disabled or diagnosed with an incurable condition. We have found, however, that no matter how severe the initial reactions, patients seem to win out over

feelings of despair. The course generally takes one to two years from
the time of occurrence or diagnosis. Those who persevere through
this phase become surprisingly well adapted to their new state of
health and ability. Social embarrassment diminishes greatly and,
even if it persists, we rarely see patients who allow it to impede them
in pursuing an active life socially or professionally. Many look back
on the initial phase of their illness and wonder why their despair or
embarrassment was so great at the time.

What advice do we have for those newly diagnosed with ST?
Simply this. Persevere. Be patient but persistent as you go through
the medical system. Specialists experienced in treating your condition may be few in your location, but once under their management,
you will find significant relief with current treatment options.
Unlike some neurologic disorders, ST is not an inexorably disabling
condition. Your pain and your outward symptoms will almost certainly improve with medical management, and your self-confidence
and outlook will do likewise.

2

Diagnosis, Coping, and Life with ST
by Nancy Muller

Little did I know that a slight head tilt to the right would eventually put me on a lifetime course that would turn my world upside down. I was thrown into a world of doctors, tests, surgery, injections, medications, coping, denial, and finally acceptance—emotionally, socially, and physically. I had a slight head tilt to the right for many years, but never thought anything of it. I had a number of medical problems through the years, one being severe vertigo. After I suffered for 19 years with it, the vertigo was diagnosed as an inner ear condition, and I had two surgeries to correct the problem. About three weeks after the second surgery, I started to suffer from severe neck pain and found myself holding my head up with my shoulder. Thus began my journey down the long road of living and coping with ST.

Symptoms of ST can start off being quite subtle, as they were in my case, with a slight head tilt and no pain at all. Normally, the onset of ST generally comes on slowly or intermittently and is usually noticed when you try to keep your head straight. There are various degrees of onset, which can include pain, twisting, tremor, and stiffness. The symptoms are enhanced with physical and/or emotional stress.

Through my experience, I've noted the importance of a proper diagnosis by a qualified neurologist with a specialty in movement disorders. For the most part, internists, family/general physicians, and orthopedic surgeons do not recognize the disease, and it often goes on for years being either undiagnosed or misdiagnosed. I was very fortunate because I worked in the medical field and was able to be diagnosed right away by a neurologist who recognized the disorder. The first step in the right direction of being able to cope with ST is proper diagnosis. I was referred to a university facility and enrolled in a research program for botulinum toxin, which at the time I was diagnosed, botulinum toxin was still in its research phase and not yet approved by the FDA.

In today's world of managed care medicine, it is difficult to make sure you are seeing the right doctors to get appropriate treatment. Insurers want to save money; they prefer treatment by primary physicians rather than by specialists. Referrals to specialists must be pushed for. The treatment of ST is highly specialized and, in order to get favorable results from treatment, the doctor needs to be familiar with the disorder so that proper treatment can be initiated.

Do research in your area as to who treats the disorder and also who is proficient in treating movement disorders. Don't take no for an answer from the insurance company; you have the right to appeal a decision, and with tenacity you can "beat the system" and receive the proper treatment. I have had to do this on a number of occasions, and have been relentless until I was satisfied the treatment I was getting was to my satisfaction.

A very important aspect of dealing with ST is the ability to accept that you have the disorder and to be able to adjust your lifestyle appropriately. Life most definitely goes on after diagnosis and you *can* live normally and productively, but you have to accept the hand that's been dealt to you and make the best of what you have. A positive attitude is a must and keeping active is a plus.

One very positive step forward is to seek out a support group in your area; if there isn't one, start your own. That's exactly what I did when I was diagnosed. I was lucky to have a doctor who was sensitive to my needs, and he suggested that I become involved in a support group. He gave me the name and phone number of such a group, but since it was too far away and met on a night I couldn't attend, I started my own. I found that the self-satisfaction of helping others made a big difference in coping with the disorder myself. If you have a computer, the Internet provides numerous resources for organizations that have support groups and also bulletin boards with great information for coping with ST from firsthand perspectives.

After being diagnosed and starting treatment, there is a period of adjustment regarding medications and possible lifestyle changes. I have worked as a full-time Registered Radiologic Technologist and back office nurse in orthopedics for 20 years. I had to make a few adjustments to make my working environment more comfortable for me but, for the most part, I could do everything I ever did before having ST. It's a matter of modifying activities in a way that reduce neck strain, such as using a natural keyboard on the computer, and using a headset when I have to spend a lot of time on the phone. I am also deaf in one ear which makes phone work even more difficult, so a headset made all the difference in the world. I have writer's cramp and found that the "natural" keyboard made typing a lot easier than on a straight keyboard. A comfortable chair with a high back could be very helpful if you do a lot of computer or phone work. Some chairs are built with a neck rest or headrest. Even the types of pens and pencils you use can make a difference in how well you can perform your job. Usually, large barreled pens with rubber grips help cut down fatigue and cramping in your hand.

I made sure to take breaks whenever I could and I'd go outside and walk for 10 or 15 minutes to loosen up and basically clear my head. One important thing to remember at work is that you have nothing to be ashamed of if your neck is distorted and/or has tremor. You have to keep up your self-esteem, as you are the same person you were before ST. I have found that if you explain what is going on to people, they are more receptive and understanding than if you say nothing. Just have a positive attitude and remember to hold your head up high (no pun intended of course!).

It is a good idea to have a neck pack at work that you can heat in a microwave. This is excellent for neck pain, as the moist heat relaxes the muscles. If you can't use it at your desk, make sure you use it at your lunchtime and breaks. I have several different kinds, like the "Bed Buddy" and some gel-filled packs. They can be purchased at most malls, and they have aromatic scents to them, along with different sizes and shapes. I prefer the packs filled with gravel-like material rather than gel packs because they provide moist heat and keep warm a lot longer.

Learn to pace yourself at work, and try not to overdo it. Easier said than done, but wearing yourself down makes the symptoms worse. Know what your limits are. Let your employer know what accommodations you require to make your job adaptable so that you can be more productive. There are specific laws governing employers through the Americans with Disabilities Act (ADA) that require them to provide needed accommodations to employees with disabilities, to allow them to perform their duties.

Another important aspect of living and coping with ST is how to act and react socially. Unfortunately when a person is "disfigured" in any way physically, it can also change him or her emotionally. This is something that you must try to overcome, because it can intensify your symptoms needlessly. There are many different directions to go for help. My number one lifesaver was the support group I started and the interaction of other groups. Talking to other people with ST helped me immensely to be able to better understand and cope with my own problems. It also helped my family learn how to support me and made them realize that they are not alone in their feelings. Being a caregiver or family member dealing with ST is a roller coaster ride for everyone concerned.

One story I clearly recall involved my own situation when I was first diagnosed, and my husband's reactions to interacting with other people with ST. When I asked him to go to a luncheon with me that happened to be a fundraiser for people with ST, he immediately found a dozen reasons not to go. He said, "I'll drive you there and pick you up, but I'm not staying." Unfortunately, he assumed there would be a whole roomful of people all twisted, tremoring, and disfigured, and he didn't think he could deal with it. I had already met with others with ST and knew that they all pretty much looked like me and weren't all twisted up like a pretzel. The stigma attached to various diseases paints such an ugly picture, and that's the mindset the average person perceives. I eventually convinced him to come with me to the luncheon, and he was pleasantly surprised at what he saw. We had a wonderful time and made some life-long friends. He met the spouses and family members of other people with ST, and they were able to discuss their own feelings and what it's like to deal with the disorder from the perspective of the caregiver. To this day, he reminds me of that situation so that I can pass the word on to others—not to judge anyone before knowing all the facts.

I feel it's very important to get out in the public and enjoy the things that make you happy. Being active is important both physically and mentally. Do whatever you feel you can do comfortably. Going out and playing golf, learning to line dance, and going to the gym are all within the limits of what you're capable of doing. Go for walks, go shopping, go to the movies, out to dinner, and any activities that let you interact with others. If you have a positive attitude about the disorder, so will everyone else around you.

I found a few years ago that playing golf was a real plus in my life, because I got outdoors and walked, I was around a lot of people, and it's a sport that makes you focus on something other than your sore neck and how you look. It turned out I can't drive the ball worth beans, but I'm an excellent putter. At the end of about nine holes, I realized I didn't have any pain at all while playing. Of course, probably because I was so focused on that silly little ball and the competitive side of me to beat my husband, I was not having any pain at all.

Another thing you might do to help yourself personally is *journaling*. This refers to daily writing down your feelings and perceptions. It allows you to express, in writing, your feelings, frustrations, and personal triumphs. Sometimes it's difficult to be able to vent to your spouse, a friend, or even a psychiatrist or psychologist. Expressing your feelings can help you to realize and gain a new perception of the circumstances that occurred. It reduces depression and anxiety of one's symptoms, and it is believed that the reduction of internal stress benefits and reduces the symptoms of ST. It's also kind of a neat way to have a record and share these things at a support group meeting. So you not only help yourself, but others can benefit from it.

I was treated for many years with botulinum toxin injections, and this significantly improved my condition and my life. Eventually, the injections were not enough, and a surgical procedure called *selective peripheral denervation* was recommended (see Chapter 7). In 1999 I had this surgery because all conservative treatments failed and nothing seem to control my pain. This surgery is very individualized, and you must realize it's not for everyone. I was very fortunate in that I had a very good result from surgery. My head was actually brought back to midline, from being tilted to the right and very shifted to the left. I was even able to bypass botulinum toxin injections for nearly a year. I am now three years post-operation and still doing better than I was before surgery. I have been back on botulinum toxin for a few years now, but I feel the surgery was worth going through for the results I did get.

Over the past year, I have entered into a different stage of my life and the disease process. I have always been very active in all aspects of my life, being a member of the workforce, volunteering my time for people with ST, recently going back to obtain a degree, and just overall always being on the go. Of course for the last few years, I've been in denial that I can still do everything I've done over the years, and twice as good to boot. This past year my health has taken a different course, and my doctors have informed me it's time to slow down and cut out all the strenuous activities I've always been be a part of. It was suggested that I file for permanent disability and start to take life easier. It took me a good year to finally come to the realization that I can't do all that I used to do, and that it's time to take it a bit easier.

At present I have filed for disability, but have been turned down on the first round. This is a whole new ball game of learning to cope all over again with a new stage of my life, and a whole new set of problems and adjustments. I have not worked for a year now, and have found that there is also a whole lot of quality to life, being able to devote myself to many of the things I couldn't while I was still working. My husband, my family, and most of all I myself know I have lots of time to devote to people with ST. My lifelong dream has been to tour the country and educate the medical profession and general public about this disorder. I plan to make ST a part of everyone's vocabulary just like cancer, AIDS, Parkinson's disease, diabetes, and other diseases that have well known spokespersons there to help them fight the battle. I plan to do all I can to help all of us with ST, so that someday there will be a cure, and I'll be able to say I was a part of it all.

So, you see, there is most definitely life after ST. It is most certainly not a death sentence, and we can all live a good life and help others do the same. To me the key to living and coping with this disorder is a positive attitude. Many researchers are trying to find the cause and cure; there are so many more alternatives as far as treatment than there were many years ago, and we have to be thankful for what we have and work with it. Don't despair: get out there in the world, be a productive member of society, and get involved. Have the self-satisfaction of not only helping yourself, but all the hundreds of thousands of people who have been diagnosed with ST and all those waiting to be diagnosed because they haven't received proper care. Let's all get involved and we *can* win the battle with ST!

3

Anatomy and Physiology

Before we get into details about the causes and mechanics of ST, we'll need some basic lessons on how muscles and joints work and how they are controlled by the nervous system.

MUSCLES AND JOINTS

We'll use a simple model to illustrate the lesson. Think of your elbow joint, which works very much like a simple hinge. The major muscle that bends the elbow is the *biceps*. In the relaxed position, the biceps is loose and elongated (Figure 2). When you want to move your arm, the motor system in your brain sends electrical signals through your spinal cord to motor nerves that terminate in the biceps muscle. When the biceps receives these signals, it becomes electrically "excited." Excitation causes the muscle to contract, shortening its lengthwise measurement, and thus exerting a pulling force on the arm bones to which it is attached on either end. Since your upper arm bone is fixed at the shoulder, this force causes your elbow to bend, drawing your forearm and hand toward your shoulder (Figure 3).

Unless you are deeply asleep, all of the muscles in your body, including those in your neck, are in a low-level state of electrical excitation and contraction, known as *resting tone*. The resting tone is determined unconsciously by constant, low-level signals from the motor system in your brain. Resting tone allows you to maintain your body posture and balance, and keeps your muscles ready for volitional action when the need arises. Your brain constantly adjusts the resting tone of your muscles depending on whether you are sitting, standing, or lying down, and how alert you are. In order to make these adjustments, your brain relies on input information (feedback) received from sensory nerve endings in muscles and

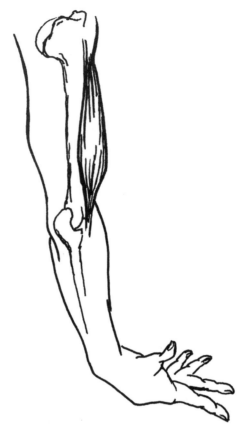

Figure 2 *Biceps muscle relaxed at full length.*

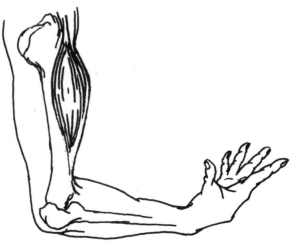

Figure 3 *Biceps muscle contracted and shortened.*

joints (including those in your neck), from the balance mechanisms in your ears, and from visual information received through your eyes. It is interesting how neck and head position is so critically managed by the brain as part of an elaborate system that controlls visual awareness, bipedal posture, and locomotion. It is perhaps surprising that such a complex system so rarely manifests clinical problems such as ST.

MORE ON THE MOTOR SYSTEM

As previously discussed, the areas of the brain containing neurons that send out signals for movement and the pathways of these signals in the deep brain and spinal cord are part of the motor system. The brain structures that make up the motor system are further divided into two subsystems: the primary *pyramidal* motor system and the secondary *extrapyramidal* motor system. The primary motor system (Figure 4) consists of neurons in the gray matter on the surface of

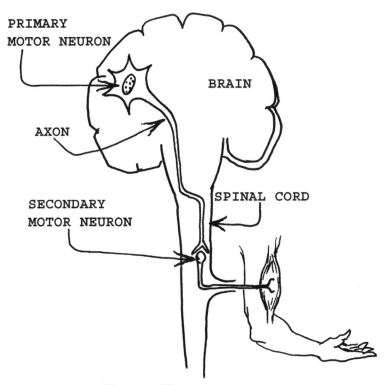

Figure 4   *The primary motor system.*

the brain's frontal lobe that send out signals for movement along wire-like processes known as *axons*. These axons run deep into the brain, through the brainstem, and down to the spinal cord, where the signals are then relayed to secondary motor neurons, which then send the signals out through their own axons to the muscles.

It would at first seem as if this primary system should be all that is needed to move your arm or any other body part, but control of movement is not so simple. You are able not only to will your arm to lift or your hand to grip, but are also able to control the distance you move your arm, the speed at which you move it, and the amount of force you exert with your arm or your grip. For example, the amount of force called for is certainly different when gripping and lifting a doughnut versus a dumbbell. The regulation of all movements and the constant minute adjustments that have to be made during movements are the responsibility of the extrapyramidal motor system.

The principal components of the extrapyramidal system are called the *basal ganglia* (Figure 5). These are a group of nut and berry-sized clusters of neurons located near the center of each half of the brain (certain of the basal ganglia together are sometimes referred to as the *striatum*). The basal ganglia receive and integrate

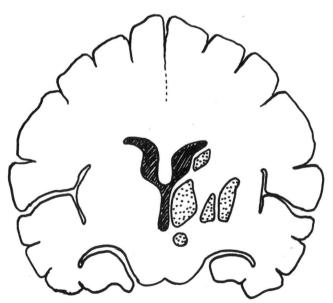

Figure 5 *The basal ganglia (stippled), part of the extrapyramidal motor system, deep in the brain.*

input information from sensory nerves and sense organs such as eyes and ears. These basal ganglia have extensive connections and interactions with the pyramidal motor system and connections to almost all other areas of the brain. The basal ganglia use sensory input information to modulate and fine-tune the output of the pyramidal motor system to allow you to accomplish tasks as different as driving a nail and threading a needle. The basal ganglia are paramount in regulating the resting tone of muscles, as discussed previously. They also prevent excess or unwanted movements by checking uncontrolled pyramidal output. Movement disorders in general are often called *extrapyramidal disorders* or *basal ganglia disorders*.

The neurons of the basal ganglia communicate among each other and with other parts of the brain by means of their wire-like axons. The terminals of these axons release chemicals that act as messengers to the cells that receive the messages. These brain chemicals are known as *neurotransmitters*. The basal ganglia neurons use a number of different neurotransmitters, including *acetylcholine* and *dopamine*. Medical conditions or drugs that interfere with the production, storage, release, elimination, or normal action of acetylcholine or dopamine may result in movement disorders. As you can see, movement disorders can be complex. A deficiency of dopamine can result in muscular rigidity, increased resting tone, or a lack or paucity of normal movement; excessive dopamine can lead to an excess of undesired movement such as tremor, twisting, writhing, or abnormal posture. Parkinson's disease is one example of a disorder in which there is a deficiency of dopamine; movements are slow and the tone is increased in this disease. However, when dopamine is given to someone who has had Parkinson's disease for a long time, excessive movements and abnormal postures may appear, as if there were an excess of dopamine. Although dopamine is suspected to be involved in ST, the exact neurotransmitter imbalance responsible for producing the symptoms has not been defined.

It is believed that the human brain has a "set point" for the natural, neutral resting position of the head and neck, with the face pointing forward, the head and chin level, and the neck following a slight natural curve. The extrapyramidal system integrates all of the sensory input information discussed above to maintain just the right amount of balanced resting tone in the neck muscles to keep the head on an "even keel." In ST, it is believed that the normal "set point" becomes altered in the brain. This could be the result of a chemical imbalance, a physical injury, or a toxin affecting components of the motor system in the brain, especially the basal ganglia. ST might also occur as the result of some aberration of the various sensory input signals from the eyes, ears, and neck.

ANATOMY AND MECHANICS OF THE NECK

The neck is one of the most remarkably agile and flexible parts of your body, partly because it must compensate for the visual limitation of having your eyes in the front of your head. Let us look at some of the mechanics of head and neck motion. Your skull rests on top of a column of neck bones, or *vertebrae*. Each vertebra is separated from the ones above and below it by a flexible rubber-like disk. The column of vertebrae and interposed disks is called the *cervical spine* (Figure 6). You can rotate your head left or right and bend it forward or sideways. Most of the rotation occurs between the first two cervical vertebrae from the top. Bending occurs to some degree between all of them.

Several muscles connect your cervical spine with your skull, and the bones of your shoulder girdle with your cervical spine and skull.

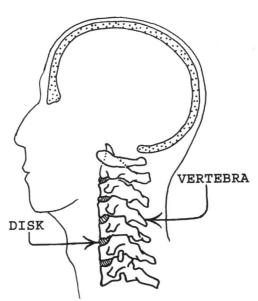

Figure 6 *The cervical spine.*

The resting tone of these muscles maintains your head and neck position. When you want to *voluntarily* move your head in any particular direction, your brain chooses an appropriate set of these muscles to contract and pull your head into the desired new position. When the "set point" becomes altered in the brain, as in ST, some muscles become involuntarily overactive.

The result is that instead of the normal balanced resting tone of neck muscles, overactive contractions of a set of muscles pulls the head and neck into an abnormal or contorted posture that approximates the new "set point." For purposes of our discussion in the rest of this book, we will refer to the primary set of overactive, involuntarily contracting muscles as *agonists*. Other neck muscles may be used, voluntarily or involuntarily, to attempt to correct head position back toward a normal resting posture. These muscles we will refer to as *antagonists*.

Depending on the particular set of agonist muscles involved, the head and neck may assume a variety of abnormal postures. The normal movement of the neck is complex, and can include forward bending (flexion), backward bending (extension), right or left turning (rotation), and right or left tilting (lateral) movements. Thus, a case of ST can be described in terms of six major directional components: *anterocollis* (flexion, Figure 7), *retrocollis* (extension, Figure 8), right or left *torticollis* (rotation, Figure 9), and right or left *lateralcollis* (tilting, Figure 10). In addition to these major directional components, ST may also involve a shifting of the head forward or backward, or to either side. In the latter case, it may appear as though the shoulder toward which the head is shifted is shorter than the other. ST may be simple, involving only one direction, or it may be complex, involving more than one component—for example, a right rotation combined with a left tilt (Figure 11). Although the word torticollis has the specific meaning of rotation, it has, through common usage, been incorporated into the more inclusive name *spasmodic torticollis*, encompassing all of the various abnormal postures.

THE MUSCLES INVOLVED IN SPASMODIC TORTICOLLIS

One of the muscles most commonly involved in ST is the *sternocleidomastoid* (SCM). This muscle stretches from the collarbone diagonally upwards along the front and side of your neck to

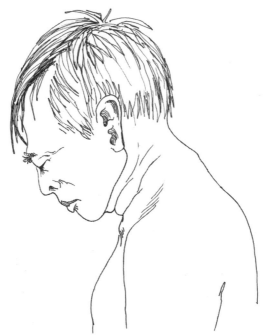

Figure 7 *Anterocollis, forward flexion.*

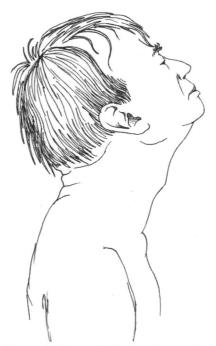

Figure 8 *Retrocollis, backwards extension.*

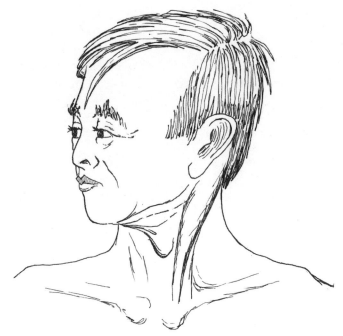

Figure 9   *Torticollis, rotation.*

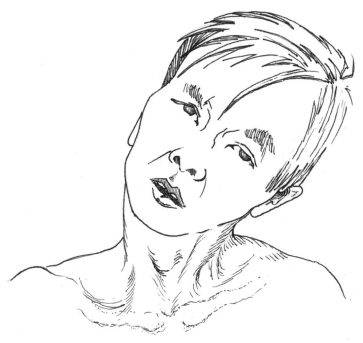

Figure 10   *Lateralcollis, tilting.*

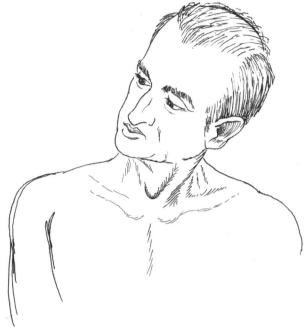

Figure 11   *Right torticollis and left tilt.*

insert on your skull just behind your ear (Figure 12). Contracting and shortening the length of your *right* SCM will rotate your face toward the *left*, while tucking your chin down toward your left collar bone (Figure 13). Contracting both of your SCM muscles will pull your head straight forward in flexion, tucking your chin into your chest. Other deeper muscles in the front of the neck are also involved in flexion.

The *trapezius* is a large, sheet-like triangular muscle that stretches from the cervical spine to the bones of the shoulder girdle (Figure 14). Contracting your right trapezius will pull the point of your right shoulder upwards and closer to your cervical spine, and also shift your head slightly to the right (Figure 15). Another muscle that raises the point of your shoulder is the *levator scapuli* (Figure 16). This muscle starts on your cervical spine and runs downward to insert along the top of your shoulder blade. It can be felt at the base, or nape, of your neck just underneath the sheet of the trapezius. You can contract both of your trapezius and both of your levator scapuli muscles if you shrug both of your shoulders upwards as if to indicate "I don't know" with body language.

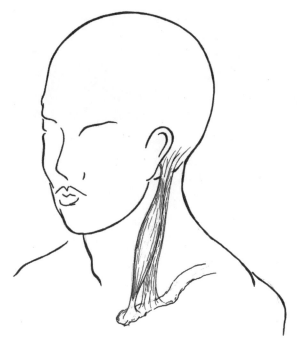

Figure 12   *The sternocleidomastoid muscle.*

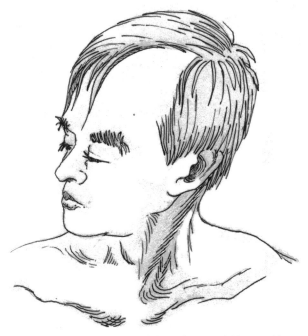

Figure 13   *The action of the right sternocleidomastoid.*

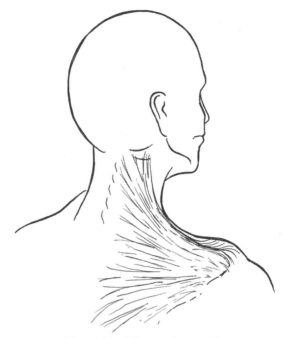

Figure 14   *The trapezius muscle.*

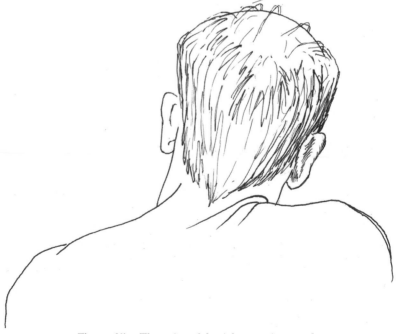

Figure 15   *The action of the right trapezius muscle.*

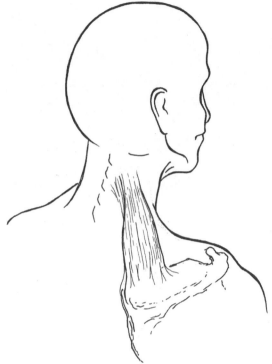

Figure 16 *The levator scapuli muscle.*

Another principal muscle is the *splenius capitis* (SC), in the back of your neck, which runs from the midline of the lower cervical spine diagonally upward to the base of your skull behind your ear (Figure 17). The pair of right and left SC muscles form a "V" in the back of the neck. The SC muscles lie in a layer underneath the broad sheet of the trapezius, which is more superficial (closer to the skin). Contracting your right SC will rotate your face toward the right, and partially tilt your head backwards in extension, moving your chin upward, away from your chest (Figure 18). Contracting both SC muscles will pull your head straight backwards in extension (Figure 19). Other muscles, lying deeper to the SC, such as the semispinalis capitis and splenius cervicis, also contribute to neck extension.

The *scalenes* are a smaller set of muscles running vertically at the side of your neck, between the back edge of your SCM and the forward edge of your levator scapuli (Figure 20). The scalenes can be seen in some thin people, but are often difficult to find. Along with

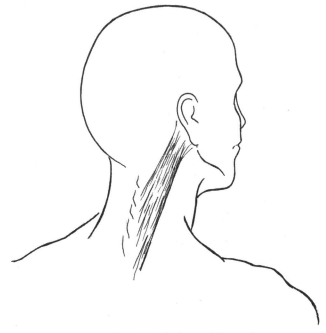

Figure 17 *The splenius capitis muscle.*

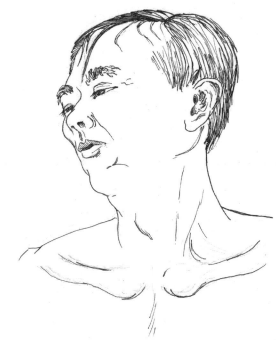

Figure 18 *The action of the right splenius capitis muscle.*

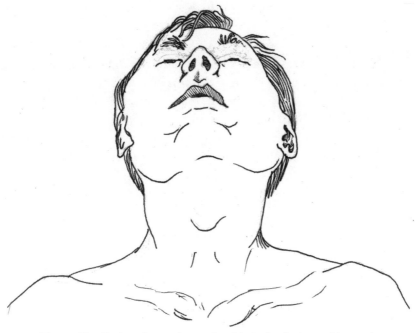

Figure 19   *Backward extension produced by both splenius capitis muscles and other posterior cervical muscles.*

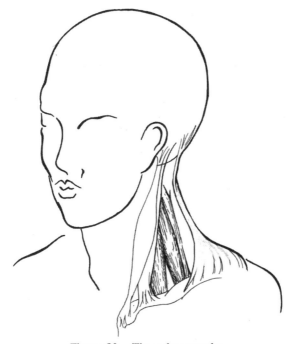

Figure 20   *The scalene muscles.*

muscles such as the SCM and others, they tilt your head sideways, bringing your ear toward your shoulder (Figure 10).

The sets of muscles we have just discussed are the principal ones involved in most cases of ST. Many smaller or deeper muscles also play a part. As previously discussed, there are six primary directions in which your head moves: flexion, extension, right or left rotation, and right or left tilting. Most torticollis patients do not have just one abnormally contracting agonist muscle. They also do not commonly have a "pure" anterocollis, retrocollis, or torticollis. Usually, a set of several muscles is overactive, producing a complex head and neck posture; for example, a left torticollis with a right lateralcollis and a slight retrocollis, a posture resulting mainly from the actions of the right SCM and left SC (Figure 21).

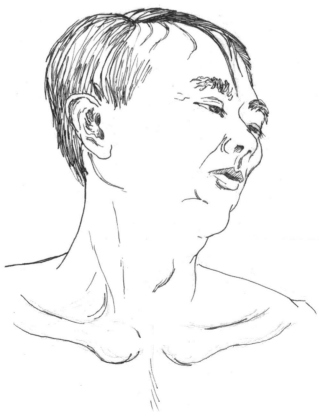

Figure 21   *The actions of right sternocleidomastoid and left splenius capitis muscles.*

PAIN

Pain deserves detailed consideration as a symptom of ST, and we can discuss the generation of pain in ST more thoroughly now that we've learned some anatomy and have a common vocabulary. Pain, along with the social embarrassment discussed previously, is one of the "hidden symptoms" in ST patients. While abnormal head posture or tremor is obvious to other people, pain is not. The incessant continuous muscle contractions in ST result in severe fatigue, producing pain in the involved muscles. This pain resembles what many of us have experienced during a "charley horse" cramp in the leg or foot. It can also resemble the muscle soreness that occurs after we perform exercise to which we are not accustomed. Such pain and soreness are temporary conditions for most people, but they are chronic (continuous) in people with ST.

Pain is generated by a number of mechanisms. The bones, joints, ligaments, muscles, and other tissues of your neck all have sensory nerve endings that send input signals, including pain impulses, centrally to the spinal cord and thence to the basal ganglia and other sensory portions of your brain. Chronic spasmodic contraction of a muscle stimulates the sensory nerve endings within it. Chronic torsion of joints, ligaments, and other tissues creates shearing and stretching forces in some places, and squeezing or compression in others. This also stimulates nerve endings in those areas. Additionally, the chronic torsional forces can hasten the development of arthritic changes in the joints between vertebral bones. Some arthritic changes involve overgrowth of bone at the edges of joints, which may then impinge on nerves entering or exiting the cervical spine.

The rubbery disks interposed between each of the cervical vertebrae can also become affected. Abnormalities of these discs are more common in ST sufferers than in otherwise healthy people. The discs can become compressed or flattened. At the same time, the edges of the discs can bulge outward into the central spinal canal. If the bulging is severe, it can compress the motor and sensory nerves attached to the spinal cord, especially if there is also bony arthritic overgrowth in the area. Spinal nerve root impingement is called *radiculopathy*, and it is likely to cause *radicular pain* that radiates outward toward the shoulder or arm. If motor nerves become severely compressed, those shoulder and arm muscles that they supply may become weak or shrunken (atrophied), leading to loss of ability to use the arm. Extreme disc bulging can even narrow the central canal and impinge on the spinal cord.

All of these factors combine to create pain. The severity of pain experienced by ST patients varies widely and does not always correspond to the severity of the abnormal position. Pain also tends to worsen with fatigue or after physical exertion. For many people with ST, pain is just as disabling, if not more disabling, as the abnormal head posture or tremor. Fortunately, severe radicular pain, muscle atrophy, and spinal cord impingement only occur in severe cases.

Chronic pain is a serious condition. It can hamper your concentration at work and at any other task. It can destroy your motivation to perform all of those activities that you need to do to live your life and also those that you perform to enjoy life. Chronic pain can create a state of apathy and even lead to clinical depression.

Fortunately, treatments that alleviate spasmodic muscle contraction and improve head position also alleviate pain. Pain responds well to chemodenervation by injection of botulinum toxin, as will be discussed later. In addition, other methods both conventional and non-conventional may be used to manage pain; these are discussed in Chapter 8.

4

The Causes of Spasmodic Torticollis

PRIMARY SPASMODIC TORTICOLLIS

It is not known why the extrapyramidal system goes awry and produces ST. The majority of cases of ST are *idiopathic,* meaning that they arise spontaneously in an individual with no identifiable cause or precipitating event. The ST is primary, meaning that it is not caused by another medical condition.

Idiopathic ST usually begins after 45 years of age. People with idiopathic ST are those most likely (about one in five) to have a spontaneous remission. The younger the age at onset of ST, the higher the chance for spontaneous remission. Remissions usually last for a few years, even a decade in some cases. Unfortunately, the permanent disorder will ultimately reemerge in almost everyone with remission. The geste antagoniste works best for idiopathic ST patients, and they tend to have longer and better honeymoon periods during the day. Placing the head or neck on a rest tends to relieve their symptoms. Their dystonia tends to remain limited to the head and neck muscles. Neck pain is mild or moderate in severity. Most individuals are able to maintain employment and normal, active lifestyles. The various medical treatments for ST tend to work best in this group of patients.

A small percentage of primary ST cases have an inherited or genetic component. Inherited forms of dystonia usually begin in childhood and tend to involve the entire body. Such inherited dystonia is often referred to as *Oppenheim's dystonia.* Family members of the affected child may also have torticollis or some other form of dystonia. Other inherited cases of torticollis begin later in life, around 50 years of age, and tend to remain focal (localized to the head and neck).

■

CASE 2

Grace first noticed some discomfort in her neck when she was 55 years of age. She was unable to maintain a neutral head position and would feel more comfortable with her head laid back while reading, watching television, or driving. She had difficulty reading, with her head pulling upwards while she read. She also noticed that her head kept moving on the pillow. Her head gradually began to pull to the right, with her chin rising, and she wasn't able to turn her head to the left easily. When her head became continually turned to the right, she developed pain in the neck and shoulder blade as well as headaches. She discovered her geste antagoniste; she found that placing her right hand on the right side of her face helped her to turn her head left. She later noted that her head turning was made worse after repetitive activity. Recently she has developed a "shaky" quality to her voice, which worsens with prolonged talking or singing high notes. Her older sister experienced similar problems two years earlier. This led Grace to seek treatment for ST. Several of Grace's family members suffer from dystonias. Two brothers and one older sister have been diagnosed with ST, and her mother and uncle had symptoms of head tremor and neck turning. Among her five children, the youngest son suffers from ST. Fortunately, Grace and her sister, who are both receiving treatment for ST, have had good responses and are now able to maintain a neutral head position.

SECONDARY SPASMODIC TORTICOLLIS

In addition to idiopathic and genetic causes, there are a number of ways by which dystonia affecting the neck may be acquired, in which case it is considered *secondary* to another primary causative factor.

Drug-Induced

The most common acquired cause of dystonia affecting the neck is a complication of certain medications. Most medications that produce movement disorders have the pharmaceutical action of blocking, augmenting, or otherwise altering the activity of the brain chemical *dopamine*. Such medications include antinausea drugs such as Compazine® (prochlorperazine) or Reglan® (metaclopramide). These dopamine-blocking medications are sometimes given intravenously to cancer patients, who may suffer severe nausea and vomiting as a side-effect of chemotherapy. Large doses of antinausea medications given at any time may produce acute dystonia or dyskinesia in any body part or in the whole body. Such acute reactions are usually transient and can usually be resolved by reducing or discontinuing the causative medication. (In rare cases, antinausea medications also may produce long-lasting [tardive] dystonias, as discussed below.) Acute dystonias can also be ameliorated with doses of Benadryl® (diphenhydramine) or Artane® (trihexphenidyl). Temporary acute dyskinesia can also occur in some patients with advanced Parkinson's disease who require large doses of dopamine-enhancing medications.

Dystonia and dyskinesias can also develop as a permanent disorder after long-term use of dopamine-blocking medications. Certain psychiatric patients require long-term treatment with medications known as *neuroleptics* or *antipsychotics* in order to remain active and functional outside of a psychiatric institution. Chronic use of these medications may result in the occurrence of late-onset, or *tardive*, dystonia or dyskinesia. This may be one reason that ST is often perceived as a psychiatric condition, since anyone who has seen residents of a psychiatric long-term care facility will be familiar with the appearance of tardive movement disorders.

It is important to note that the most commonly used psychiatric medications are antidepressants such as Elavil® (amitryptiline), Prozac® (fluoxetine), Paxil® (paroxetine), or Zoloft® (sertraline). These medicines are not dopamine-blocking agents and are not associated with the development of tardive dystonias.

Both acute and tardive drug-induced dystonias and dyskinesias are neurologic movement disorders that involve abnormal signals from the brain that cause the spasmodic contraction of a set of muscles and result in abnormal posture. When they affect the neck, the resulting syndrome is similar to ST, although there is a greater tendency to have backward jerking of the head. Unfortunately, the tardive syndromes are chronic or permanent conditions. After first reducing or eliminating the causative medications, tardive movement disorders may be treated by the same methods as primary ST; however, they do not respond as well to these treatments. Fortunately, newer generation neuroleptics have a much lower tendency to produce such side-effects, so drug-induced movement disorders are becoming less common.

Brain Damage

Brain damage suffered during fetal development in the womb or during infancy or early childhood may predispose an individual to develop dystonia later in life. Such early damage may be the result of complications of pregnancy or birth that cause oxygen deprivation (*anoxia*). It could also be caused by fetal jaundice, in which toxins from the breakdown of blood cells and from liver dysfunction accumulate in the basal ganglia of the brain; or by an early brain infection (*encephalitis*), caused by bacteria, viruses, or certain parasites.

Any cause of respiratory or breathing failure in adulthood may result in brain damage and dystonia if the resulting oxygen deprivation, or anoxia, is severe enough to cause prolonged loss of consciousness or coma. Such anoxia may occur during a heart attack, if rescuers are unable to resuscitate the victim quickly. Anoxia may also result from a drug overdose that depresses breathing. Such overdoses may occur accidentally during recreational drug abuse, or intentionally in a failed suicide attempt. Near-drowning or suffocation is another cause of anoxia. Anoxia has a predilection for harming components of the extrapyramidal system, including the basal ganglia. However, most sufferers of anoxic brain damage do not have isolated dystonia, but also have other neurologic deficits.

A severe blow to the head that is sufficient to produce coma for a length of time may result in a number of neurologic deficits, including dystonia. In these cases, dystonia does not occur as an isolated disorder. Such people almost always have memory problems, impairment of understanding and communicating in verbal or written language, other cognitive deficits, incoordination of movements, or even a paresis (lack of movement) of body parts in addition to dystonia. A single concussive blow to the head that only produces dizziness, or even transient loss of consciousness, will not produce dystonia.

Stroke

A stroke occurs as a result of the plugging, or *occlusion*, of a brain artery, leading to the death of neurons and other brain cells in the territory supplied by that artery. Alternatively, a stroke may occur because of rupture and blood leakage from an artery. Occasionally, strokes that involve the basal ganglia or other parts of the extrapyramidal system will result in dystonias and possibly ST. Only a small fraction of all strokes affect the extrapyramidal system in this way. A much larger percentage of strokes affect the primary pyramidal motor system, resulting in muscular weakness (*paresis* or *paralysis*) in the affected body part. True muscle weakness of this type is not a feature of dystonia.

Toxins

Medications that alter the activity of the brain chemical dopamine may produce a permanent tardive dystonia that closely resembles ST. These medications have been discussed above. Other environmental toxins are also known to produce movement disorders that can resemble ST. For example, the metallic element manganese has produced movement disorders among those who mine its ore, and mercury or lead contamination from industrial sources can also cause movement disorder symptoms, its other effects. Fortunately, with governmental regulations and better industrial safety practices, such cases have become much less common.

Medical Disorders

Medical disorders that usually affect other parts of the body may produce movement disorders if the brain becomes involved. One such disorder is *systemic lupus erythmatosus*, also known as SLE, or just lupus. In this disorder, the immune system begins to attack normal body tissues, including those of blood vessels in the brain and the brain tissue itself. Other such medical conditions include *Sydenham's chorea*, a later complication of rheumatic heart disease; *Wilson's disease*, a complication of the body's inability to utilize the essential mineral copper; and some inborn problems with metabolizing certain nutrients. Almost all of these medical conditions produce a variety of physical signs and symptoms that distinguish them from idiopathic ST.

Physical Injury to the Neck

Physical injury, or *trauma*, deserves special discussion as a cause of ST. Physical brain injury producing torticollis has been discussed above, and it is usually accompanied by a number of other neurologic impairments. What we will discuss here is the onset of ST after *peripheral* trauma, usually to the neck. We must at this point also exclude those neck injury patients who have sustained orthopedic injury to the cervical spine, causing a dislocation or fracture of any of the vertebrae. In the early 1990s, one of the authors of this book reported a small number of trauma-induced ST cases in the medical literature. These patients shared many similar characteristics, which are typified in the description of trauma-induced ST given below. Since this first report, other cases have been described.

Typically, individuals who develop trauma-induced ST have a mild to moderate neck trauma from falling, being struck in the neck, or suddenly catching or lifting a heavy object. Sometimes they have had a "whiplash" type injury. They sometimes report hearing a "snap" or "crack" at the time of the injury. Typically, they begin having neck pain and a feeling of stiffness immediately afterwards. Within weeks to a few months, they begin to develop abnormal neck posture, most often a lateral tilting toward one shoulder, and continued or increased pain. X-rays and other imaging studies do not reveal the fracture or dislocation of any neck bones.

In comparison to people with idiopathic ST, trauma-induced ST patients often don't experience any relief of symptoms with head rest or support. The geste antagoniste is not as effective in relieving their symptoms. Pain is a more severe component of their disorder. Medical treatments for ST do not work as well for these individuals as for those with the idiopathic disorder. In particular, treatment with botulinum toxin, described in Chapter 7, does not work as well. A greater percentage of them become limited in their activities or disabled and unable to work.

The importance of trauma as a causative factor in ST has been debated in the neurologic community for many years and remains a point of controversy. There are convincing arguments that some degree of sudden neck strain or minor trauma occurs frequently in the lives of active people, and that when one of them develops ST, there is a tendency to want to attribute it to an external cause. The issue is further complicated because many people who claim a traumatic cause are involved in litigation over the trauma and its resulting after-effects.

Neck trauma, whiplash, and similar injuries are common events. Certainly, only a tiny fraction of all such injuries results in the development of ST. It is not clear why a very few people who sustain such a trauma develop ST while the vast majority do not. Some among this small number may have a genetic predisposition to develop movement disorders. It is also not clear how a relatively minor neck trauma can induce changes in the basal ganglia and extrapyramidal motor output of the brain to result in ST. It may be that the trauma disrupts the normal sensory inputs from muscles and joints of the neck to the brain and thus changes the information the brain uses to maintain its "set point" for head position.

We can say that, among the hundreds of dystonia patients seen in our clinic over the years, we have identified only a handful who appear to have ST caused by trauma. In those cases that we have identified, ST symptoms began within days of the injury. Given that almost all of us have experienced a number of falls, tumbles, or neck strains at different times in our lives, there is no way to know whether an injury in the remote past has resulted in ST for any individual.

CASE 3

Jake was 20 years of age when he was working in the tire industry. One day while lifting a large truck tire, he felt an abrupt pain in his neck. He immediately noticed that his neck was turned to the right, with his head tilted towards his right shoulder. He was unable to turn his head, and when he needed to look to the left, he had to turn his whole body in that direction. Because the pain in his neck was so severe, he went to a chiropractor and had physical therapy, which included massage and wearing some form of a harness that was designed to help straighten out his neck. He had no significant improvement with these treatments. He continued to work in a warehouse, however, managing as best as he could in an attempt to prevent total disability. Jake saw many doctors as well. He was once diagnosed as having Parkinson's disease, but the medications prescribed for Parkinson's disease did not work for him. This disorder had a major emotional impact on Jake's life. He had practically no social contact and only one date in 27 years. He started drinking alcohol in an attempt to help alleviate his pain and became an alcoholic. Twenty-seven years after the onset, Jake consulted a neurologist who specialized in ST and was subsequently treated with injections of botulinum toxin. His life was changed. This was the first time he experienced some pain relief. He stopped drinking alcohol, became more socially involved, and eventually married.

5

How Is Spasmodic Torticollis Diagnosed?

The diagnosis of ST is fairly difficult compared to other medical conditions. For instance, when a person contracts pneumonia, he or she has fairly specific symptoms that include coughing, fever, and malaise. The doctor, who may have seen hundreds of cases of pneumonia, recognizes the condition by listening to the lungs with a stethoscope and performing other diagnostic tests to confirm the diagnosis and direct treatment. An X-ray will show fluid in the lungs, and a sputum culture will allow identification of the bacteria causing the infection, thereby directing the choice of antibiotic.

In contrast, the symptoms of ST can be caused by a number of other conditions, including "wry neck," or neck muscle strain. ST is a rare disorder as medical illnesses go. It is estimated that only about three people out of 10,000 have some degree of ST. A primary care physician may thus only see one case of ST in several years, and that may be a mild case that is not easily recognized. Couple this with the fact that most patients walking into a doctor's office with a cocked head and neck pain are actually suffering from transient wry neck or one of the orthopedic or other neurologic disorders that mimics ST. Such a patient may, appropriately, receive treatment with analgesic pain medications, muscle relaxant medications, heat, ice, massage, physical therapy, or even chiropractic care. In many mild cases, these conservative measures alone may make the symptoms tolerable or acceptable, even if the definitive diagnosis of ST is not made.

There is no blood test, other laboratory test, or imaging study that will diagnose ST. The abnormality affecting the basal ganglia in ST is chemical or functional in nature. It is, therefore, not visible on conventional brain imaging studies such as *computed tomography* (CT) or *magnetic resonance imaging* (MRI). The diagnosis is made when a neurologically experienced physician obtains a detailed history from the patient regarding the onset and progression of the

41

symptoms, and then performs a careful physical exam. For these reasons, many times a person suffering from ST may not receive the appropriate diagnosis the first time he or she is seen by a doctor. Often, a person with ST will be seen and treated by many different doctors for many years before receiving the appropriate diagnosis.

■

CASE 4

Helen was 35 years of age when she began to notice pain in the left side of her neck and back of her head. She thought she was having headaches and treated herself with over-the-counter medications such as aspirin and ibuprofen. The pain was constant and she noticed she was most comfortable in positions in which her head was supported. Over-the-counter medications did not help much and she sought help from her primary care physician. She was given various pain medications. Because her head tilted towards the left shoulder and her left shoulder was elevated, her doctor prescribed physical therapy for muscular strain. Neither the medications nor the physical therapy helped the pain she felt in her neck, head, and left shoulder. She developed stomach problems due to the pain medications. Because of the pain, she was unable to continue working and lost her job in a department store. She became depressed over this and mentioned it to her doctor, who referred her to a psychiatrist. The psychiatrist gave her antidepressant medication and, although her mood improved, the pain in her neck did not. She then was referred to a pain specialist who gave her nerve block injections and even destroyed one of the nerves thought to be causing her pain. The pain continued. She finally was diagnosed with ST when she was referred to a neurologist for treatment of her continuing headaches.

If conservative measures do not work, the patient may be referred to an orthopedic specialist. Those patients who have orthopedic causes can then receive the appropriate treatment. Certain patients suspected of having exposure to psychiatric medications may be referred to a psychiatrist. In fact, people with drug-induced dystonia of the neck are probably more common overall in the medical setting than true primary ST patients. This is probably the reason that ST is perceived as a psychiatric illness, or that ST patients are presumed to have an underlying psychiatric disorder.

Whether a true ST patient is initially referred to an orthopedist or psychiatrist, he or she should eventually be suspected of having a neurologic disorder and be referred to a neurologist. It is usually a neurologist who makes the definitive diagnosis. Most neurologists have enough experience with ST and other dystonias to recognize the disorder and initiate treatment. Even in a general neurology practice, however, ST cases make up only a tiny fraction of the patient population.

Whether a neurologist provides more advanced treatment for ST depends on the concentration of his or her practice. Therefore, a neurologist will sometimes refer patients who do not respond well to treatment, or those who have severe or complicated cases, to a sub-specialist in the field of movement disorders. Neurology clinics specializing in movement disorders are mostly found at major university medical centers, although some neurologists specializing in move-ment disorders practice at private medical centers, in private groups, or independently in the community. Appendix A will help you to locate such specialists.

During the interview, the physician will try to ascertain the presence of factors in your medical history known to cause movement disorders. These might include a history of birth complications that can result in brain injury. Other historical factors include brain infection during infancy or later, previous head injury affecting the brain, or a known history of stroke. Any event during which the brain is deprived of oxygen (*anoxia*) at any point in a person's life may produce dystonias. Such episodes may include near-drowning, smoke or fume inhalation, choking or other causes of asphyxiation, cardiac failure such as occurs during a heart attack, or the pro-longed respiratory failure that can occur in drug overdoses. In order to produce a permanent movement disorder, the anoxia must be severe enough and prolonged enough to produce coma for some length of time.

It is especially important for the diagnosing physician to know if the patient has ever been admitted to a psychiatric facility, has been under any psychiatric care, has received chronic treatment for gas-trointestinal disorders of nausea or dysmotility, or has otherwise been exposed to neuroleptic medicines. In our practice, past exposure to neuroleptic drugs is the single most common cause of a neurologic condition that looks almost identical to primary ST. Some examples of medications that can cause such disorders are Haldol®, Thorazine®, Stellazine®, and Reglan®.

If other causes of dystonia are not found during the interview, the physician should suspect the presence of an idiopathic movement disorder, and he will then examine you thoroughly. He may first want to establish the presence of over-contracting or spasming muscles in the neck by looking carefully for their bulging and also by feeling the relative firmness or flaccidity of various muscles. Experienced physicians can often tell by carefully observing head position and direction of tremor movement, and by sense of touch, exactly which particular neck muscles are primarily involved in the ST.

The physician will usually perform a more generalized neurologic exam to look for coexisting conditions or dystonic involvement of other body parts. He may look for problems in memory and cognitive abilities, disorders affecting the pyramidal motor system, spinal cord problems, and dystonia affecting any of the limbs, face, eye closure muscles, or voice. He may order laboratory tests to screen for some of the medical disorders discussed previously that can produce dystonia.

Depending on the presence of certain factors in your medical history or findings on the physical exam, the physician may order X-ray study, CT scan, or MRI of the neck to ascertain the presence of an orthopedic abnormality in the cervical spine. A brain imaging study, usually an MRI, may be indicated if there is a history of stroke or head trauma. As previously discussed, the basal ganglia abnormalities that produce ST are not visible on MRI. Once other conditions are eliminated by history, physical examination, and any indicated tests, the definitive diagnosis of idiopathic ST may be made.

OTHER CERVICAL CONDITIONS

Spasmodic torticollis, the neurological movement disorder, needs to be distinguished from a number of other neck conditions, some of which produce abnormal posture.

Tension Cervicalgia

The most common condition confused with ST is sometimes called "wry-neck," although this term has been loosely used for a variety of conditions, including ST. Wry neck is usually a result of an acute neck muscle spasm or strain-producing pain. Nearly everyone at some time has awoken one morning with a new neck pain, or a "crick" in the neck. A person so affected may *intentionally* hold his or her head in a position so as to minimize the pain, or may be reluctant to turn the head normally to look in a different direction. Instead, he or she may turn his or her entire body to look in a particular direction, giving the appearance of a "stiff" neck. We prefer to use the term "tension cervicalgia" to refer to this condition. We prefer not to use the term "wry-neck" at all, since its meaning is ambiguous. Tension cervicalgia usually abates with conservative treatments such as stretching, massage, posture correction, and simple analgesics.

Orthopedic Conditions

As discussed above, ST is a neurologic disorder, with the pathological process occurring mainly in the motor system of the CNS. A number of muscular and skeletal conditions may resemble ST. One such condition is *atlanto-axial dislocation,* a slippage of the top two bones of the vertebral column, which occurs as a result of physical injury. Some children are born with one or more neck muscles shortened, otherwise poorly formed, or missing altogether, creating a tethering effect that results in malposition of the head and a restricted range of neck motion.

These muscular and skeletal conditions fall under the realm of orthopedics rather than neurology. They can mimic the appearance of ST, but are not caused by abnormal signals from the CNS producing dystonic contractions of a set of muscles. Orthopedic conditions will not respond to the treatments used for neurologic ST; they are usually treated with physical therapy, splints, collars, or surgery. There is extensive literature on various forms of orthopedic torticollis affecting infants and young children, but these conditions will not be discussed in this book.

NEUROLOGIC CONDITIONS

A number of other neurologic conditions may have ST as one of their manifestations. Most common among these are drug-induced conditions. Some medicines used to treat nausea and vomiting, and certain psychiatric medicines called *neuroleptics* or *antipsychotics,* may produce acute transient dystonia or dyskinesia as a side effect. Prolonged treatment with such medications can produce a permanent movement disorder, called *tardive dyskinesia*, that closely resembles ST and persists after the medication has been stopped. This is probably the reason that torticollis is often perceived as a psychiatric condition. It should be stressed that the movement disorder is not a result of the psychiatric illness, but a complication of the medications used to treat it. Drug-induced movement disorders are discussed in more detail in Chapter 4.

OTHER DYSTONIAS, DYSKINESIAS, AND MOVEMENT DISORDERS

Within the realm of neurology, movement disorders comprise a wide variety of conditions. Dystonias and dyskinesias can involve any part of the body and can occasionally be *diffuse*, involving the face, neck, trunk, and all four limbs. They may occur as isolated conditions, or may coexist with ST or with each other in any individual. Some individuals may start out with symptoms of ST, then begin to experience symptoms of another dystonia at a later date. Dystonia starting in one body part may spread to the neck. Some people with ST have family members affected by another dystonia. For these reasons, we discuss commonly seen dystonias below.

Writer's Cramp and Focal Limb Dystonias

Some focal dystonias have symptoms that only occur when an individual is performing a certain action or activity. *Writer's cramp* develops most often as an idiopathic disorder. The individual experiences an involuntary contraction of hand, wrist, or forearm muscles that impairs writing with a pen or pencil. Depending on the particular muscles involved, the writing instrument may become gripped more tightly, dropped out of the hand, or held at an odd angle that makes penmanship impossible. The wrist can uncontrollably flex or extend upwards. The fingers may contort into odd positions.

Writer's cramp almost always begins in the hand most used for writing. In the beginning, symptoms may only manifest after writing an entire page or more. As the condition progresses, the dystonia becomes disruptive after only one sentence or word. It may even become difficult for the individual to sign his or her name.

Depending on their job, some individuals (such as doctors) need to do a great deal of handwriting on a daily basis. Unfortunately, over time, writer's cramp tends to progress fastest in those who attempt to continue writing. A similar disorder is seen among musicians who perform intricate finger movements on their instruments, such as violinists or pianists. Odd focal dystonias have been described among people who perform intricate repetitive motions with their hands, such as soap wrapping or parts assembly. Tremor and dystonia of the hands may persist even when the specific activity is not being performed. Such disorders are collectively called *occupational dystonias.*

Writer's cramp and occupational dystonias respond poorly to most medical treatment. Medications used for dystonia have only moderate effect. Chemodenervation injections with botulinum toxin provide moderate relief, often allowing individuals to continue to use handwriting or finger play as is necessary for their employment. Unfortunately, although botulinum toxin injection alleviates symptoms and somewhat improves performance with the hands, it does not improve the underlying brain abnormality or remove the causative repetitive motion. If affected individuals continue to perform the causative activity, such as continuing to write frequently, their disorder may progress until other activities, such as combing the hair or using eating utensils, also become impaired. Occasionally, if the unaffected hand is used as a substitute, it too will become affected over time. Our advice to such patients is to limit the causative activity as much as possible. Writer's cramp patients whom we treat are advised to keep handwriting to a minimum and to use a keyboard or laptop computer as much as possible. However, in some individuals, the disorder may begin to occur when using the keyboard or even when performing unrelated activities.

Spasmodic Dysphonia

Spasmodic dysphonia is an idiopathic dystonia that is even more rare than ST. The pitch and sound of a person's voice is controlled by a pair of muscular vocal cords located in the voice box, or larynx. One set of muscles, the *adductors*, pulls the cords closer together; another set of muscles, the *abductors*, pulls them apart. Dystonia affecting either or both sets of these muscles can result in impairment of the voice.

Adductor spasmodic dysphonia gives a strained quality to the voice, as if the person were trying to speak while being choked. The voice is quiet, and it is difficult to produce loud speech. If more severe, the voice is characterized by irregular, choppy silences caused by intermittent stoppage of airflow. *Abductor spasmodic dysphonia*, with the vocal cords pulled apart, results in a breathy, whispering quality to the voice and is not characterized by stoppages. Adductor dysphonia is the more common form. Sometimes, both forms coexist in the same patient, creating a mixture of symptoms.

Neurologic spasmodic dysphonia must be distinguished from a number of other throat conditions that produce hoarseness of the voice. Most such disorders do not produce restriction or change in airflow. The most common among these is inflammation of vocal cords, which may be due to an infection such as laryngitis, or due to irritation from the chronic reflux of stomach acid.

Spasmodic dysphonia can occur as an isolated disorder, or it may coexist with other dystonias, especially those involving face and neck muscles. It often coexists with ST. Spasmodic dysphonia may be so mild as to not be noticed or diagnosed, or it may become severe enough to be socially or professionally disabling. Although it responds poorly to oral medications, it does respond well to injections of botulinum toxin into the dystonic laryngeal muscles. Laryngeal botulinum toxin injection is a highly specialized procedure, usually performed only by experienced neurologists or ENT (ear, nose, and throat) physicians.

Facial Dystonias

Blepharospasm is an idiopathic involuntary squinting or complete closure of the eye. This is caused by dystonia of the *orbicularis oculi*, a thin disk of muscle that lies just beneath the skin and completely encircles each eye socket. When it contracts, the orbicularis oculi works in a manner similar to a camera shutter and squeezes the upper and lower lids of the eye together. You can see this camera-like action if you slowly squeeze one eye tightly shut while standing in front of a mirror. Blepharospasm may occur on one side only, but most often affects both eyes. If the spasm becomes frequent or prolonged enough, the disorder can be disabling. Blepharospasm responds well to botulinum toxin injections into the orbicularis oculi, having relatively few complications.

Oromandibular dystonia can involve the tongue or other muscles of the mouth and jaws. There are three different forms. The most common is a form in which the jaws are clenched together, closing the mouth forcefully. Such patients may involuntarily grind their teeth, damaging them or any dental work. In another form of the dystonia, the jaws are held apart and the mouth is open; patients have great difficulty in keeping it closed. In another form, the lower jaw is forcefully displaced sideways. Oromandibular dystonia may also involve face muscles, causing lip pursing or "kissing" movements. The tongue may move in different directions, sometimes involuntarily thrusting out of the mouth. A combination of lip movements and tongue movements, accompanied by dystonia of other facial muscles, may be referred to as *Meige syndrome*.

Oromandibular dyskinesia is most frequently seen among psychiatric patients who have been treated with dopamine-blocking psychiatric medications. If the face and lip muscles are involved, the patient may make repetitive "munching" movements resembling the snout movements of rabbits. They may also make lip pursing or "kissing" movements.

Oromandibular dystonia or dyskinesia can be extremely disfiguring, socially crippling, and painful. Tongue and lip movements may interfere with speech. They can be difficult to treat, even with well-placed botulinum toxin injections. The mouth-closing form responds best to treatment while the other two forms do not respond as well. Interestingly, a "sensory trick" such as placing a toothpick in the mouth or a menthol candy on the tongue can temporarily reduce the dystonia and improve speech.

Others

Generalized dystonia is, fortunately, a rare condition. It usually begins as a focal dystonia, but then progresses over a period of months or years to involve most of the spine, trunk, and limbs. This is a disabling condition and is one of the inherited forms of dystonia beginning in childhood. Affected individuals have a great deal of difficulty in maintaining employment. Depending on the eventual severity of the condition, they may become unable to care for themselves independently, and even become bedridden in extreme cases. Genetics research has shown that some people with this disorder have an abnormality in a specific gene that is passed on to half of their offspring, although not all of those who receive the gene develop dystonia symptoms. botulinum toxin injections can be used to alleviate the dystonia in a specific area, usually the neck. However, because of the widespread muscle involvement, even maximum doses of botulinum toxin do not improve their functional ability or significantly improve their condition. The best that can be done is to manage such patients with high doses of one or more oral medications, pain management, and supportive care. Permanently implanted pumps that deliver medications such as baclofen directly into the spinal column have been of benefit to some patients.

Hemifacial spasm is an intermittent or continuous contraction of muscles on one side of the face. It is often mistakenly called a *tic*, but tics are another type of neurologic entity that can produce facial twitching. The distinction may be difficult to make, even for an experienced neurologist. Hemifacial spasm is usually caused by compression of the facial motor nerve by a blood vessel. It results in pulling on one side of the mouth, often with intermittent squinting of one eye. If face muscle contraction is strong enough, the pulling force may produce a slight head tremor. While not disabling, hemifacial spasm may cause unacceptable disfigurement or social impediment. Botulinum toxin injections to facial muscles alleviate the disorder, but the resulting weakness of treated muscles may cause a temporary asymmetry of facial expressions such as smiling.

6

Pharmacologic Treatments

There is no cure for ST. Those cases that are secondary to medications, even tardive dystonia, may improve with time after discontinuation of the causative agent. For ST, there are only treatments to alleviate the symptoms. However, this improvement is significant in most cases. There are basically three major modes of medical treatment for ST: oral medications, injection of a muscle-weakening agent, and surgery. This chapter mainly discusses the oral medications used to treat ST. We will discuss each of the different pharmaceutical classes of medications that are used. Within each of these classes, those individual drugs that are commonly used will be mentioned. We will then discuss the general principles and strategy of medication management. Treatment with injections and surgery is discussed in the next chapter. Every patient and every case of ST is different, and thus the treatment plan appropriate for your case needs to be developed by your treating physician with your cooperation.

ORAL MEDICATIONS

Until the early 1990s, this was almost the only medical treatment applied to ST. Overall, oral medications have limited usefulness in ST, and these medications have changed very little in the past 20 years. The common medications used for ST can be divided into pharmaceutical classes, each of which shares common mechanisms of action and, for the most part, a common group of side effects. These general characteristics are discussed for each class, accompanied by a listing of several commonly used medications within each.

Anticholinergics

Anticholinergic medications all act by suppressing the effects of the *parasympathetic* nervous system, a part of the nervous system that controls a number of involuntary automatic functions in our bodies. These include the formation of tears and saliva, the motions of the intestines that propel digested material forward, heart rate, the storage and release of urine, and the responses of sex organs. The major chemical by which parasympathetic nerves send their messages to their target organ, such as a salivary gland, is *acetylcholine*, and medications that suppress the effects of parasympathetic signals are called *anticholinergics*.

If you were to be given *excess* acetylcholine, or a drug that *increases* the effects of acetylcholine, you might become sweaty, salivate or drool, have watery eyes, and feel intestinal cramps or the need to defecate or urinate. The side effects of *anticholinergic* medications are the opposite: you may feel hot and dry on your skin, experience dry or "cotton" mouth, and have constipation or even difficulty emptying your bladder. Additional side effects at higher doses of medications can include drowsiness and mental confusion. Fortunately, if doses of medications are started at low levels and then increased gradually, your body can become accustomed to the change in parasympathetic activity, and the side effects will usually diminish and become easily tolerable.

Two commonly employed anticholinergic medications are Artane® (trihexphenidyl) and Cogentin® (benztropine mesylate). Either of these medications is sometimes given to psychiatric patients together with each dose of their neuroleptic medication, in order to prevent the onset of acute or tardive dystonia. These medications need to be taken three or four times each day. The doses of anticholinergic medication for ST may be six or seven times higher than the recommended doses for other disorders for which these medications are used. The low starting doses rarely provide benefit for ST. Slow increases over time, under the supervision of a physician who monitors side effects, are required to achieve the high doses needed to obtain benefit. At high doses, these medications provide mild to moderate relief of the muscle spasms and head twisting, although they are not very effective at relieving pain. If you are currently using one of these medications and are not experiencing severe side effects, there are a few precautions you should take. You should stay out of extreme heat, as these medications reduce the ability to sweat, and you should drink plenty of fluids to counteract dry mouth and constipation. If you are having difficulty urinating while on these medications, consult your doctor.

Sedatives

Most sedative medications used for the treatment of ST fall into a family of drugs known as benzodiazepines. The benzodiazepines most commonly used for ST are Valium® (diazepam) and Ativan® (lorazepam), although Klonopin® (clonazepam) is used for ST and some other neurologic disorders. Other benzodiazepines include Xanax® (alprazolam), Librium® (chlordiazepoxide), Restoril® (temazepam), and Halcion® (triazolam). Benzodiazepines are most commonly used in low doses as anxiety relieving medications. They are also sometimes used as prescription sleeping aids. At higher doses, they may be used to treat epileptic seizures or to calm severely agitated or violent patients.

It is not known exactly how benzodiazepines improve dystonia, but they do have a muscle relaxing effect. It is known that they enhance the activity of the inhibitory brain chemical *gamma aminobutyric acid* (GABA). This may diminish the abnormal motor signals coming from some group of neurons within the extrapyramidal system. There may be other mechanisms by which benzodiazepines exert their effects. It is not likely that the therapeutic effect of benzodiazepines on ST symptoms is due to their effects as sedatives. ST patients do experience some drowsiness when initially started on benzodiazepines, but they soon become accustomed to this effect. Symptom relief tends to persist even as drowsiness diminishes. The muscle spasm–relaxing effect of benzodiazepines is most likely responsible for the sustained therapeutic effect.

As discussed above, sedation is the major side effect of benzodiazepines. Drowsiness in the evening is usually not a problem, but daytime drowsiness can be bothersome. For some reason, however, the ST patients for whom we prescribe these drugs tend not to feel their sedating side effects as strongly as people for whom these medications are prescribed for other reasons. We do not know why ST patients are more tolerant of this side effect, but it is lucky that they are, since the doses required for control of ST symptoms are much higher than doses required for anxiety control. At extremely high doses, incoordination of the limbs can occur.

One major concern patients have about being prescribed benzodiazepines is their potential to cause drug addiction. They may have heard of the names of some commonly used benzodiazepines as drugs that are used by drug abusers. When it occurs, addiction usually happens to patients taking the drugs for other diagnoses, such as anxiety disorder or behavior control. Addiction is very uncommon among dystonia patients. In fact, we have yet to see true addiction and abuse of benzodiazepines in any of our ST patients.

An important distinction must be made here. *Addiction* is not the same as *dependence*. If a medication does what it is supposed to do and significantly reduces ST symptoms, then a patient may depend on it to function normally. Additionally, once the patient's motor system and brain have adapted to a certain dose of benzodiazepines, the medication should not be stopped abruptly. Abrupt discontinuation of medication may result in temporary worsening of symptoms (*rebound effect*), and other withdrawal symptoms such as seizures may occur. Benzodiazepines can be discontinued in any ST patient who desires it, but this should be done by a gradual dose reduction over a few weeks.

The list of benzodiazepines is extensive, and the choice of which one to use is best made by your treating physician. We usually choose to prescribe Valium®, mostly because we are familiar and comfortable with dosing it. The major difference between various benzodiazepines is the speed with which they are absorbed after swallowing and the number of hours their effect lasts. In general, drugs that are absorbed and take effect quickly will last for a shorter length of time, and vice versa. Overall, high doses of benzodiazepines provide mild to moderate relief of ST symptoms.

Antispasticity Medications

These medications are most often used to treat muscle spasticity that occurs in disorders of the primary, or *pyramidal*, motor system, such as strokes and spinal cord injuries. There are differences in the type of increased muscle tone seen in pyramidal motor system disorders versus extrapyramidal movement disorders, but these differences need not concern us at this point.

The first antispasticity medicine is baclofen. It has the effect of enhancing the activity of the brain chemical GABA. GABA is widely distributed in the brain and spinal cord, and has an overall inhibitory effect on the motor system. Increasing GABA activity thus tends to keep runaway motor output signals in check. Baclofen is most frequently used in spinal cord injury patients who have spastic or "jumpy" legs, but it can provide some improvement for dystonia patients. The major side effect is sedation. The authors' experience shows that it has only a mild beneficial effect for ST, but the side effect is fairly easy to tolerate. There is no addiction potential, but abrupt discontinuation can result in a temporary rebound increase in spasticity symptoms, so discontinuation must be done gradually.

Two other antispasticity medications belong to a family of drugs called *alpha receptor agonists*. The details of alpha receptor functions need not be discussed here. The exact way in which these reduce muscle spasms is not well defined. The two most common of these medications are Catapress® (clonidine) and Zanaflex® (tizanidine). Catapress® is used most often as a blood pressure-lowering agent. Zanaflex® is used for muscle spasticity, to relieve muscle pain of the type associated with tension cervicalgia and a condition known as *fibromyalgia*. Both are used for pyramidal spasticity and may be applied to extrapyramidal dystonias. The major side effects are sedation and low blood pressure, which may cause light-headedness when standing up. Zanaflex® tends to relieve some pain associated with dystonias. In our experience, these two medicines provide minimal benefit to ST patients at tolerable doses; side effects usually limit the use of higher doses.

Another antispasticity medicine is Dantrium® (dantrolene). This medication works within the cells of muscle tissue, inhibiting the contraction of those cells and thereby the contraction of the entire muscle. Doses of Dantrium® high enough to diminish muscle spasms usually cause diffuse weakness in all the muscles of the body and usually produce sedation as well. For these reasons it is rarely employed for the treatment of focal dystonias such as ST, and our own experiences in prescribing it have not yielded very impressive results.

Dopamine-Enhancing Medications

Dopamine-enhancing medications work in a number of ways to increase the activity of dopamine in the extrapyramidal motor system. They are most often used to treat Parkinson's disease, in which dopamine-producing neurons of the extrapyramidal system stop functioning and eventually die. Sinemet® is a commonly used Parkinson's disease medication that delivers a chemical called *levodopa* to the brain. Levodopa is subsequently converted to dopamine. Other medications, called *dopamine agonists*, deliver to the brain chemicals that behave very much like dopamine and have similar effects. Dopamine agonists include Mirapex® (pramipexole), Requip® (ropinirole), Permax® (pergolide), and Parlodel® (bromocriptine).

There are a small number of dystonia patients whose symptoms are alleviated by the dopamine-enhancing drugs used for Parkinson's disease. In fact, these patients are sometimes said to have "*dopamine-responsive dystonia.*" Dopamine-responsive dystonia is one of the inherited forms of dystonia. The side effects of dopamine-enhancing medications are fairly mild compared with those of other classes of medications discussed in this chapter. These side effects include nausea, loss of appetite, sedation, and constipation. Side effects at higher doses may include hallucinations and even transient acute dyskinesias. These usually only occur in patients with more advanced Parkinson's disease; most other patients tolerate all of the side effects quite well. Dopamine-enhancing medications should be tried for a brief period of time in appropriately selected ST patients. Unfortunately, only a tiny fraction of patients have a dopamine-responsive dystonia.

Antidepressants

Medications in this class have a variety of different mechanisms of action. They are, of course, used to treat depression. If an ST or dystonia patient also has associated depression, his or her doctor may choose to employ a medication from this class. Many of these medications have anticholinergic side effects, providing some relief from dystonia as well, though this benefit is smaller than that achieved with true anticholinergics. Apart from these effects, however, antidepressant medications have the property of reducing the symptoms of chronic pain, which is a frequent sequela of ST. The mechanism by which these medications relieve chronic pain is not known. However, because of this property, they are sometimes used to alleviate chronic headaches as well as the pain from pinched nerves or other disorders of the peripheral nerves.

Side effects of antidepressants vary with the type used. The most frequently experienced side effect is sedation. Anticholinergic side effects such as dry-mouth, constipation, and urinary retention are also experienced. The most commonly used antidepressants for pain belong to a family known as *tricyclic* antidepressants. These include Elavil® (amitriptyline), Tofranil® (imipramine), and Pamelor® (nortriptyline). Tricyclic antidepressants may be the most effective for pain control, but they have greater side effects. Other newer antidepressants, called *selective serotonin reuptake inhibitors*, or SSRIs, have fewer side effects, and their pain-relieving properties are still being elucidated. These include Zoloft® (sertralene), Paxil® (paroxetine), and Celexa® (citalopram).

THE STRATEGY OF ORAL MEDICATION THERAPY

As you have no doubt gleaned from reading the preceding sections, all of the medications used for ST seem to have limited benefit. Although a few people have an excellent response to one or more medications, with great improvement of symptoms, the vast majority experiences only a mild or moderate relief of neck twisting and pain. Additionally, as you have no doubt noticed, most of the medications have significant side effects. If your doctor decides to try oral medications to treat your condition, he will choose a medication from the class best suited for you in terms of the severity of your condition and the presence of any other conditions that may require treatment. For example, in the presence of depression or significant nerve pain, an antidepressant medication may be the best choice for a first try. A brief trial of dopamine-enhancing medication may be appropriate for certain patients to avoid missing a case of dopamine-responsive dystonia. All other things being equal, anticholinergics and benzodiazepines are the most frequently chosen medications to treat ST.

Regardless of which medication is chosen, the motto for dosing is "start low and go slow." This means that the starting dose should be low enough to avoid intolerable side effects. The dose is usually increased slowly over a number of weeks, while the doctor and the patient monitor the occurrence and severity of side effects. Increasing the dose gradually allows the body to become used to the drug and to compensate for side effects. For example, the anticholinergic effect of dry mouth tends to diminish with time. The sedating side effects of many medications also diminish, allowing higher doses to be used.

The biggest reason many patients "fail" a medication trial is that they do not see any improvement in symptoms after the first few weeks. During this time, they may experience some side effects and then stop taking the drug. The initial low dose may not be enough to improve symptoms, but may cause some side effects. In general, it may take several weeks or even a few months of therapy to find out if a particular drug is going to be of any benefit. Our biggest concern in oral medication therapy is that a particular drug has been declared ineffective, when, in fact, an adequate trial of appropriate duration and dose has not been done. If the first medication tried is not effective or is not tolerated, a second choice must be made and the process started again. Remember, ST is a chronic, usually life-long condition. It takes a great deal of patience and perseverance on the part of you and your doctor to find the most beneficial medication and dose.

PAIN CONTROL

Pain has been discussed as an integral component of ST that can be more disabling than the abnormal head posture, and we previously referred to it as one of the "hidden symptoms" of ST. The alleviation of pain is of paramount importance in treating ST patients and is thus discussed separately in detail. Pain responds well to treatment with botulinum toxin, discussed in Chapter 7. Medications used to treat the spasming muscles, usually Artane®, Valium®, or other benzodiazepines, also alleviate pain. However, supplementary treatments often are needed specifically for the pain.

First-line pain medications include anti-inflammatory analgesics, either in nonprescription or prescription strength. We generally choose ibuprofen (Advil®, Motrin®, others), or naproxen sodium (Aleve®, Naprox®, others). These medications are also our first choices for relieving any local injection site pain that may occur after botulinum toxin injections. As adjuncts to these, we may add medications that contain a narcotic analgesic substance, such as Vicodin®, which contains hydrocodone. The list of medications that contain hydrocodone or a similar narcotic is long. We try to not prescribe narcotic pain medications on an "as needed" basis because the risks of both narcotic dependence and addiction are fairly high. We have noted that our ST patients who receive such medications have difficulty in discontinuing them.

For patients with persistent focal pain in one or two particular areas, injection of a local anesthetic agent to those tender or "trigger" points can alleviate pain on a temporary basis. Lidocaine and bupivicaine are the most commonly used local anesthetic agents. Such local anesthetic injections, also referred to as "trigger point" injections, may be effectively used to keep pain at a tolerable level between scheduled chemodenervation treatments (discussed in Chapter 7), which are usually about three months apart.

7

Chemodenervation and Surgery

As you have learned, oral medications have limited benefit in ST patients and are difficult to use because of side effects. Fortunately, there is another way to reduce the over-contraction of agonist muscles pulling on the head and neck. The injection of a muscle-weakening agent into the muscles of the neck can normalize the head posture, relieve spasms, and reduce pain. Surgery can be employed to cut nerves or muscles involved in the torticollis. We will first discuss the injection of muscle weakening agents, a procedure known as *chemodenervation.* Various surgical procedures will then be discussed.

CHEMODENERVATION AGENTS

Chemodenervation agents work by disrupting motor nerve endings within a muscle. The muscle then cannot receive the signal to contract. The treated muscle becomes loose, slackened, or paralyzed for a prolonged period of time. We will begin by discussing the development of chemodenervation agents and their application to ST patients.

Formerly, solvent chemicals such as *phenol* were used for chemodenervation. Although phenol still has useful applications, the agent most frequently used now is *botulinum toxin.* Botulinum toxin is produced by the species of bacteria called *Clostridium botulinum. C. botulinum* is present in the environment in an inactive form. It is an *anaerobic* bacterium, meaning that it thrives in environments devoid of oxygen. Such an environment can be found inside a can of preserved food or in the depths of a puncture wound in human tissue. If the inactive *C. botulinum* contaminates such an environment, it can become active and flourish, resulting in a spoiled can of food or an infected wound. When it becomes active, the bacterium releases a toxin that is poisonous to nerve endings. In humans, this poisoning is a disease known as *botulism*, a complication of dirty, infected wounds or the eating of certain spoiled foods. People with botulism become progressively weaker in all parts of their body, as muscles become progressively loose, flaccid, and paralyzed; ultimately, the person can no longer move. In most cases, muscles of breathing become affected and, unless the patient is given artificial respiration, the disease will be fatal. When placed on a respirator, the patient can be sustained until nerve endings regenerate, a process that may take several months.

Botulinum toxin certainly sounds like a frightening substance to employ for medical therapy. Indeed, botulinum toxin was first isolated and purified from the bacterium more than 50 years ago as a part of experiments to find potential biological weapons for the United States military! However, during the 1970s, the toxin was purified from bacteria cultures grown in a laboratory and then carefully processed for injection into muscle tissue for therapeutic medical use.

Purified botulinum toxin was first employed to treat a disorder of the eyes called *strabismus*, in which the two eyes are misaligned with one another. When injected into appropriate muscles behind the eyeball, it can correct this misalignment. It soon became apparent that botulinum toxin could be used to treat almost any medical condition that is characterized by increased muscle tone or abnormal muscle contraction in any part of the body. Dystonias and dyskinesias are primary among such disorders.

There are several strains, or subspecies, of *C. botulinum*, each of which produces its own variation of botulinum toxin. The different types of botulinum toxin are classified according to their chemical structure. Toxin type A is marketed in the United States under the brand name of Botox®, and toxin type B under the name Myobloc™. Other types are available outside the United States, including Dysport®, a formulation of toxin type A. Botox® and Dysport® are supplied as dried crystals of toxin in a vacuum container and have to be diluted with saline prior to injection. Myobloc™ is supplied already diluted in liquid form. As of this writing, Dysport® is only available in the United States under research protocols.

INJECTION OF BOTULINUM TOXIN

The first step in chemodenervation treatment is to determine which muscles need to be targeted for injection. Your doctor does this by first observing the position and movement of your head. From her knowledge of the anatomy and normal movement actions of various muscles, she can reasonably guess which muscles are involved. Sometimes, long over-contracting agonists can be visibly bulging in the neck or even have become enlarged from the prolonged exercise much in the same way as a weight lifter's muscles become enlarged. Your doctor may then examine the muscles by *palpation*, touching and pressing them to confirm which are abnormally contracting.

In some cases, this is all that is necessary to establish the target muscles. In other cases, the target muscles may not be so obvious, and diagnostic testing may be necessary. Diagnostic testing usually consists of *electromyography* (EMG) in which an electrically conductive needle is inserted into a suspect muscle, and the electrical output of its muscle cells is recorded. After several muscles on each side of the neck are tested, the doctor has a "map" of the most active muscles contributing to the abnormal head posture.

The next step is to determine the dose of botulinum toxin to be given to each muscle and the overall dose to be used for a particular patient. There is no set dose for each muscle or for any patient, although there are some rule-of-thumb guidelines. Larger muscles require higher doses than smaller muscles, and strongly contracting muscles require higher doses than moderately contracting ones. Additionally, the overall dose is determined by the physical size and muscularity of the patient. A large, athletically built man will certainly require much more toxin than a slim, petite female. If too little toxin is given, there will be little beneficial effect, and any reduction of the symptoms will be short-lived. If excessive toxin is given, neck muscles may become too weak, and the patient may have difficulty keeping his or her head upright. For these reasons, our practice is to start off with a mid-range or conservative dose. Although this may not provide maximum benefit, it allows us to assess how the patient responds to the treatment and safeguards against possible side effects.

Another complication in deciding the correct dose is that the measured units are not the same among the three formulations of botulinum toxin. Fifty units of Myobloc™ is not equivalent to 50 units of Botox® or to 50 units of Dysport®. In the end, your doctor must choose your doses based upon the severity of your ST, the particular muscles involved, your physical size, and the particular formulation of botulinum toxin he chooses to use. Sometimes, nearby muscles that were not injected will take over the function of chemodenervated muscles, resulting in a change in the pattern of the torticollis. This will require reassessment and modification of the treatment approach. It may take several subsequent treatments with various doses and targeted muscles before an optimal response is achieved, one that is effective without causing excessive weakness or side effects.

Botulinum toxin may be injected into target muscles through a conventional hypodermic needle. In some cases, a doctor may choose to deliver the injection through an insulated electrically conductive hypodermic needle attached to an EMG machine. Simultaneous recording of EMG activity allows the doctor to know when the needle tip is exactly within the body of the target muscle. It takes approximately three days before the effects of botulinum toxin injections are noticed, and three to four weeks for maximum effect to be seen. After this, the effects begin to slowly wear off, as nerve endings within the muscles regenerate. The beneficial effect lasts for about three months, after which the injections must be repeated.

Chemodenervation by botulinum toxin injection is currently the most effective method of relieving the abnormal muscle spasms of ST. The effectiveness in any person with ST depends on the severity of his condition. Botulinum toxin never fully restores the natural resting position. For our own patients, our goal is to improve head position by 50–70%, and we select muscles and injection doses according to this goal. Fortunately, botulinum toxin is as effective, if not more effective, in ameliorating the pain component of ST as it is in improving head position. This is often more important to the person suffering from ST.

Some patients expect that their ST will continue to improve progressively with each successive treatment until the condition is completely resolved. This is unfortunately not the case. Symptoms return as the effect of botulinum toxin wears off. For instance, suppose a patient with a rotational torticollis of 60 degrees receives chemodenervation treatment and that the rotation subsequently improves to 30 degrees. As the toxin's effect wears off over time, the patient's head will slowly drift back approximately to the original 60 degrees of rotation. Subsequent chemodenervation treatments should have about the same effect as the first one, improving the rotation to approximately 30 degrees. Subsequent treatments will not progressively improve rotation until neutral position is reached.

A few patients have even noticed that the results from their first chemodenervation were the best, and that subsequent treatments did not produce the same degree of improvement. This phenomenon has many explanations, which may vary from individual to individual. Many muscles, large and small, are involved in most cases of ST; botulinum toxin is usually injected into only the largest and most accessible of them. Therefore, even in the best scenario, some residual head pulling persists. After some length of time, uninjected muscles, often smaller and deeper in the neck, may take over the lead, pulling the head back to its abnormal set point. We have seen, during neck surgery on some of our patients for whom chemodenervation treatments had become ineffective over time, that some of these deep, normally small muscles had become enlarged from the involuntary exercise. Our inability to identify such muscles (prior to surgery), or the inability to inject them without substantial risk to the patient, may account for the diminished effectiveness of subsequent chemodenervation treatments in some patients. However, an experienced physician may be able to cope with this problem by varying the injection technique to target these previously untreated muscles.

Sometimes, a patient who has had a stable level of improvement with each botulinum toxin injection will notice a loss of effectiveness after several years of treatment. This may be due to the development of antibodies that make an individual resistant to the botulinum toxin. The more frequently injections are given and the higher the toxin dose at each treatment, the greater is the tendency for an individual to develop resistance antibodies. Therefore, it is recommended that injections be given no more frequently than every three months and that the lowest effective dose be used at each treatment. Patients who develop resistance to one type of toxin may subsequently respond to injection of a different type. For example, Myobloc™ may be effective after Botox® has stopped being effective.

As with any injected medication, a local skin infection or allergic medication reaction is possible. However, sterile needles and alcohol wipes have nearly eliminated the occurrence of infection. Allergic reactions to botulinum toxin are very rare with the purified formulations currently used. Side effects from the botulinum toxin injections include local redness and slight bruising from the injection needle. Some patients experience numbness in the treated area. Difficulty with holding the head upright may occur if larger doses are required for severe ST cases. The toxin may also spread from the point of injection through tissues of the neck to the larynx, or voice box. The usual result is mild swallowing difficulty or hoarseness of the voice, requiring a soft or pureed diet for several days. Rarely, breathing difficulties can occur. Most side effects resolve over days or weeks. There is no known permanent impairment from botulinum toxin injection. Botulinum toxin injection for chemodenervation is now a principal treatment for ST, and is recommended by the American Academy of Neurology and the National Institutes of Health. Both Myobloc™ and Botox® have been approved by the FDA for the treatment of ST.

SURGICAL TREATMENT

In order to discuss surgical treatment, we will have to further discuss the anatomy of the neck. The cervical spine is depicted in Figure 6. Each vertebra of the spine is shaped like a ring, with a hole in the middle. When they are stacked together to form the cervical spine, the holes form the *central spinal canal*, through which runs the spinal cord (Figure 22). At each vertebral level, the spinal cord gives off a pair of right and left nerve roots that contain the outflow axons of neurons of the motor system. The nerve roots exit the cervical spine through gaps between the vertebrae called *foramina*. The roots may merge with each other. Either before or after merging, they branch into motor nerves that terminate in various muscles. One single nerve root may supply signals to a number of muscles, but each muscle receives its signals mainly through one single terminal motor nerve branch.

PERIPHERAL SURGERY

The spinal nerve roots are fairly easy for a surgeon to locate at the point where they exit from between the vertebrae of the cervical spine. One easy way to stop overactive agonist muscles would be to cut those nerve roots that supply them, a procedure known as *rhizotomy* (Figure 23). There are drawbacks to such an approach, how-

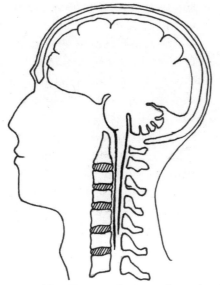

Figure 22   *The cervical spine and spinal cord.*

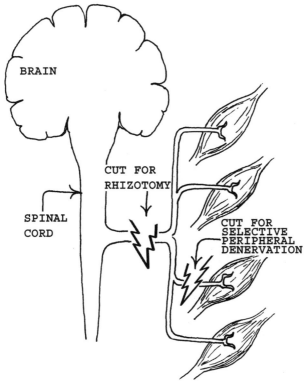

Figure 23   *Surgical sites for rhizotomy and selective peripheral denervation.*

ever. Since one root supplies several muscles, many more than just the targeted agonists would become severely weakened or paralyzed, causing excessive neck weakness. Since the surgery is permanent, there would be no way to reverse this weakness. Although there are variants of rhizotomy that involve only partial cutting of a nerve root, this procedure has largely been superseded by a technique known as *selective peripheral denervation.*

The technique of selective peripheral denervation was developed in the 1970s by Dr. Claude Betrand. It requires somewhat more finesse than the standard rhizotomy described above. In this procedure, a surgeon must locate motor nerve branches supplying the targeted agonist muscles, follow them to their termination point in the muscle, and cut them just at that point (Figure 23). Selective peripheral denervation is a highly specialized procedure; it should be performed by an experienced neurosurgeon in conjunction with a movement disorders specialist.

The muscles to be targeted must be carefully selected prior to the surgery. Sometimes, the best muscles to target are difficult to identify, even for an experienced movement disorders specialist using EMG guidance before and during the surgery. Our strategy, for some of our more complex patients, has been to first perform a partial operation, targeting only those muscles that are obviously involved. We then allow the patient to recover out of the hospital, after which we carefully reassess him to select target muscles for a second surgery. The goal is to abolish the abnormal contraction in most of the muscles producing the unwanted movement, while preserving nerve connections to adjacent normally acting muscles. Selective peripheral denervation works best for patients with rotational torticollis and least for patients with retrocollis. Physical therapy is required to recover the full range of motion of the neck following surgery.

Adverse effects from surgery include a permanent weakness of adjacent neck muscles that causes difficulty in holding up the head or in swallowing. Rarely, weakness of the diaphragm can occur, causing a breathing impairment, because the nerve that controls this muscle passes close to some target muscles. Fortunately, we have been able to substantially reduce the occurrence of these adverse effects in recent years by refinements in surgical technique. For instance, we use an electrical nerve stimulation technique that allows us to identify and cut a nerve at a point just before it enters the target muscle, well after it has already given off branches to adjacent muscles, such as those involved in swallowing. Despite all refinements, however, there are anatomic and physiologic variations among patients, and adverse events may still occur.

Another surgical procedure is called *myotomy*. Myotomy involves the cutting or removal of portions of the overactive agonist muscles. Because of the greater amount of tissue trauma from this procedure, internal scar tissue may form and adhere to adjacent muscles and ligaments, limiting the range of neck motion or causing pain. Although myotomy may still be applied in certain cases, selective peripheral denervation is becoming the surgical procedure of choice. In certain cases, the two procedures may be combined for maximum benefit.

BRAIN SURGERY

The procedures discussed above all involve surgery on peripheral nerves or muscles. Attempts have been made to treat ST and other movement disorders with surgery of the brain, specifically involving some alteration of the basal ganglia.

Thalamotomy is a technique in which a surgeon inserts a probe deep in the brain to destroy a small piece of brain tissue in the basal ganglia (see Figure 5). This destructive lesion alters the output of the extrapyramidal motor system to achieve the desired effect on a patient's symptoms. The probe must be targeted with great precision, using guidance techniques such as CT scanning and MRI. Sometimes, the result obtained after an initial operation is inadequate, but repeating the procedure with an attempt to make a larger lesion may bring further improvement. Paralysis similar to that seen in a stroke may occur if the target is missed by a fraction of an inch. Thalamotomy is permanent.

Thalamotomy has more recently been superseded by a nondestructive technique known as *deep brain stimulation*. This involves insertion of a thin electrical wire into specific targets within the basal ganglia. The wire is attached to a battery-powered device similar to a pacemaker that is implanted under the skin. Low-level electrical impulses from this device disrupt the electrical output of the basal ganglia that is causing unwanted movements. If the effects of stimulation are not desirable, the device can simply be turned off or removed if necessary.

Thalamotomy and deep brain stimulation are mainly used as treatments for advanced Parkinson's disease. They are especially useful for Parkinson's patients in whom the disease is characterized by an inordinate amount of tremor and who respond inadequately to medications. These techniques have been applied to more widespread or generalized dystonia with limited success. Unfortunately, they have not as of yet been found to be effective in ST. Experimental trials are currently underway for torticollis patients and may yield another alternative treatment for severe cases.

SPINE SURGERY

The authors have seen a small number of patients who had received cervical spine fusion surgery for the treatment of ST. Basically, this involves the harvesting of pieces of shaved bone from other parts of the body, then grafting them into place as bridges across adjacent cervical vertebral bones. The grafted pieces of bone fuse into place, locking adjacent vertebrae together into a rigid unbendable column. This may seem like a logical way to keep the head straight, but think about this: the abnormally contracting muscles will continue to exert their pulling force. The difference is that they will now exert tension and torsion forces on joints that cannot bend or give way. In our experience, this creates worse bone and muscle pain than before. In such patients, pain may become so severe that they are forced to use narcotics on a chronic basis.

We have attempted to treat such patients by chemodenervation with botulinum toxin injections or with selective peripheral denervation. However, these two treatments often fail to relieve pain symptoms in patients who have had spinal fusion. The reason for this is that not every single muscle involved in the ST can be targeted for injection or denervation, and these leftover secondary muscles continue to exert a small pulling force. Even this small residual pulling force is enough to produce pain when it is applied against a rigid, unyielding spinal column. Spinal fusion surgery may be appropriate for patients who suffer from *orthopaedic* causes of torticollis, but it is not appropriate for patients who have ST, the *neurologic* movement disorder. In our experience, we have never found spinal fusion surgery to have benefited any ST patients who have had it done. It is simply not helpful, and may be harmful.

WHO WILL BENEFIT FROM SURGERY?

All surgical procedures carry the risk of producing excessive weakness or paralysis, causing infection or internal bleeding, complications of anesthesia, or simply not being effective. In light of these considerations, how are candidates for surgery selected from among ST patients? Simply put, all nonsurgical treatments are attempted first. Surgery is never considered as a first-line or early treatment, even in fairly severe cases of dystonia, because some cases may resolve spontaneously, given time. Additionally, the specific muscles involved at the beginning may change over time. Some muscles may stop contracting and new ones may become involved. The proper muscles to target may not become obvious until the disorder stabilizes.

Chemodenervation with botulinum toxin remains the mainstay of treatment for ST, supplemented by oral medications and pain management. As discussed previously, some patients may develop resistance to botulinum toxin after years of repeated injections. Those patients for whom chemodenervation is no longer effective may be considered for surgery. Among those patients, surgery works best for those with rotational torticollis, and less well for those who predominantly have retrocollis or anterocollis. Other factors may influence a patient's suitability for surgery. The coexistence of medical conditions such as heart disease, diabetes, lung or breathing problems, or blood clotting abnormalities will add to the risk of adverse outcomes from surgery.

Selective peripheral denervation is becoming the procedure of choice for those patients who are appropriate candidates for surgery. Note that, as opposed to *surgical* denervation, the injection of phenol or botulinum toxin achieves a *chemical* denervation. Chemodenervation is not permanent, but destructive surgery is. Also, surgery of any kind rarely completely cures ST. Peripheral surgeries on the nerves and muscles do not alter the abnormality in the extrapyramidal system of the brain. The brain may recruit adjacent muscles, usually smaller and often not previously involved in the ST, into activity in order to bring the head back to its abnormal set point. Patients who undergo surgery do not usually become free from the need for continued treatment. Many of them must continue receiving botulinum toxin injections and/or medications. All of the factors discussed above must be considered together in selecting any one patient for surgery.

8

What Else Is There?

PHYSICAL THERAPY

If available, physical therapy by an experienced therapist may improve pain symptoms. The goals of physical therapy include bringing the head position back toward normal, increasing the range of motion, and decreasing pain, thereby increasing functional ability. The physical therapist may employ a variety of techniques to achieve these goals. Primarily, he will gently move the neck through its range of motion, stretching the spasming agonist muscles. He may take advantage of the effect of geste antagoniste, stimulating the skin by gentle stroking or by applying ice to decrease the contraction of agonists during neck maneuvers. For some patients, gentle neck traction using a mechanical device may alleviate pain. Physical therapy techniques such as ultrasound or diathermy also may help with pain. Neck strengthening exercises should be limited to the antagonist muscles and will be discussed in Chapter 9.

MASSAGE

While it is used extensively by some of our patients and is a fairly effective treatment for tension cervicalgia, local massage tends to have mixed results in ST. While it almost always feels good while being performed, pain control is very short-lived. In some patients, massage, especially deep massage, aggravates the spasms and contractions of agonist muscles. As a result, pain may actually *increase* following massage. However, we have found that an acupressure type treatment, in which the point of an elbow is applied to a spasming trapezius muscle, or to muscles in the back of the neck, is often beneficial. Pressure should not be applied to the sternocleidomastoid muscle, which runs along the front and side of the neck, since doing so is ineffective and may even cause injury. Overall, we have found that properly applied acupressure is a most economical and effective pain relief measure with very low risk or side effects, and it may be performed at home by a spouse or family member.

CHIROPRACTIC

Chiropractic manipulation of the neck is generally safe. It is dangerous only in a cervical spine that has been fractured, that has an unstable dislocation of one or more vertebrae; or that has arthritic changes that may predispose to damaging an important artery during manipulation, resulting in a stroke. Other than in these situations, which most chiropractors will exclude by examination and X-rays, chiropractic intervention carries minimal risk, especially with the modern safer neck manipulation techniques in wide use today. However, we find that the vocabulary employed in the chiropractic realm is not quite the same as ours. Torticollis, as diagnosed by a chiropractor, may not be exactly the same condition as the neurologic movement disorder we are discussing in this book. Additionally, treatments and techniques vary widely among chiropractors, and it is impossible for us to comment on the benefit any one patient may experience by visiting an individual chiropractor. Overall, in the medical literature, chiropractic manipulation has not been shown to be effective in alleviating either the abnormal neck posture or the pain associated with neurologic ST.

CERVICAL COLLARS

We are aware of rare patients who are able to use collars to ease their performance in specific situations. For instance, one of our patients wraps a soft collar about her neck while driving. The rubbing of the soft foam rubber against her skin provides a *geste antagoniste* that aids her in looking forward down the road. However, she does not use the collar at most other times. Cervical collars may provide a feeling of temporary relief from ST, however, they may also cause harm.

Cervical collars are intended for short-term use, and ST is usually a chronic (long-term) problem. Use of a cervical collar over a period of months may lead to weakening of the neck musculature—all muscles, not just those that are overactive. Cervical collars, especially the hard collars, rub against the back of the neck and can induce muscle spasms. Uncontrolled head motion may even cause enough rubbing against the collar to break or ulcerate the skin, especially in older patients. These effects can make the torticollis worse or increase the pain. Finally, hard collars may increase the chance of neck injury; a dislocation of the spinal bones can result from a wearer falling down the wrong way. For these reasons, we rarely recommend cervical collars in the treatment of ST.

MISCELLANEOUS

Other forms of treatment may also be helpful. Occupational therapy can help with stress management, mobility, energy conservation, and the use of adaptive equipment. Psychological counseling may help patients to understand the nature of their pain and the effects it can have on them, and techniques for coping with chronic pain can be learned. Hypnosis, while not harmful, has not been found to be useful, because ST is not primarily a psychiatric disorder.

Biofeedback, acupuncture, and acupressure are alternative treatments that may aid in pain management. A TENS (transepidermal nerve stimulator) unit, a wearable device that delivers low-level tingling electrical stimulation to the skin, can provide temporary pain relief. Your doctor may refer you to a physical therapy facility, a pain management clinic, or a practitioner who specializes in these various interventions.

WHAT CAN I DO FOR MYSELF?

Maintaining optimal health is the best way to cope with a chronic disorder such as ST. As we all know, a good healthy diet and regular cardiovascular exercise is important to achieve this goal. No vitamins, minerals, or special diets have been proven to be beneficial specifically for torticollis. Stimulants such as caffeine and nicotine may transiently aggravate torticollis symptoms; however, there is no evidence that these substances cause permanent worsening. Although alcohol can have some muscle relaxing effects and briefly improves a few movement disorders, its use is not recommended as a treatment for ST. Exercise is an important part of maintaining health, but there are a few things you should keep in mind if you have ST. It is important to maintain as much flexibility of the neck as possible. Gentle stretching exercises of the neck are recommended. You should avoid sudden manipulations or extremes of movement with respect to your neck. The concept of "no pain, no gain" does not apply here; you should let pain be your indicator to quit an exercise. Otherwise, judicious aerobic exercise is good for your cardiovascular system and maintaining optimal health.

9

Rehabilitation Exercises

SPECIFIC EXERCISES YOU CAN DO AT HOME

This chapter describes some exercises that you can perform on your own. They are specific for the treatment of ST and are designed to accomplish two major goals:

1. Stretch and relax the overactive agonist muscles that are in spasm.
2. Strengthen the antagonist muscles that can oppose the torticollis and bring the head position back to neutral.

The exercises in this chapter are designed to be used in conjunction with medical treatments such as oral medications, chemodenervation injections, physical therapy, and pain management interventions. In general, you will be applying the stretching exercises to the overactive agonist muscles in conjunction with chemodenervation. As the overactive muscles are weakened by chemodenervation, they will be easier to stretch using the above exercises. As the agonists relax and their pulling force diminishes, it will become easier to perform strengthening exercises on the opposing antagonist muscles.

The particular exercises appropriate for you will depend upon the muscles involved in your particular case of ST. Ask your treating physician to specify which of your muscles are acting as agonists. In general, these are the ones that are being injected with botulinum toxin, and you should practice those stretching exercises specific for them. Also ask your physician which antagonist muscles he would recommend for strengthening. In most cases, these will be the muscles that correspond to the agonists on the opposite side of your neck, but additional antagonists may need strengthening as well. If you have a physical therapist, he may be able to help in selecting the particular muscles and exercises that are appropriate for you.

The exercises have been designed to be performed with a bare minimum of easily obtained equipment. With a few modifications, they can be performed in almost any setting, at home or at work. All of the exercises described are to be performed slowly—you should perform all of them in slow motion. If any movement produces pain, you should stop and seek further advice from your doctor.

STRETCHING EXERCISES

The first exercises are simple stretches. Many of the following stretching exercises can be done in the standing or seated position. Most require some type of suitable handhold. In the standing position, the height of the handhold should be about the mid-thigh level, close to where the hand rests naturally. A suitable object to grasp might be a heavy table or desk. In the seated position, a sturdy chair with a suitable leg or cross bar should suffice. For some exercises requiring a handhold in front of you, the front edge of the seat may be grasped. Use a stable chair with a backrest and without wheels. The illustrations depict a common type of inexpensive metal folding chair available at most office or home warehouse stores.

Exercise one: Splenius capitis, levator scapuli, and others

This exercise is designed to stretch and relax the muscles that run down the back of your neck on either side of your neck bones, as well as the muscles that connect these bones to your shoulder blades. It may be useful for individuals who have a component of rotational torticollis plus retrocollis (as in Figure 21). It is performed in a seated position on a chair that allows you to grasp and hold underneath (Figure 24). Alternatively, it can be performed in the standing position next to an object that has a handhold at approximately the mid-thigh level. We will illustrate stretching for the left-sided muscles. The entire procedure may be reversed if you require stretching of the right-sided muscles.

Grasp the handhold with your left hand. Slowly lean your body forward and toward the right side, and at the same time allow your left shoulder to relax and be pulled downward while keeping your grip on the handhold. You may feel a pulling or stretching sensation deep in your shoulder muscles. Next, turn your head about 45 degrees toward the right, then tilt your head into a direction away

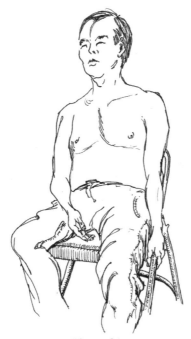

Figure 24

from your left arm. As you do this, feel the stretch in the muscles of your shoulder and the back of your neck on the left side. Hold this position for 30 seconds. You may feel the sensation of stretch begin to subside. At this point, you may actually be able to stretch a little further. To make the stretch even more effective, reach over the top of your head with your right hand and gently help pull along the direction of the stretch (Figure 25). Hold this position for another 10 seconds, then slowly release and relax.

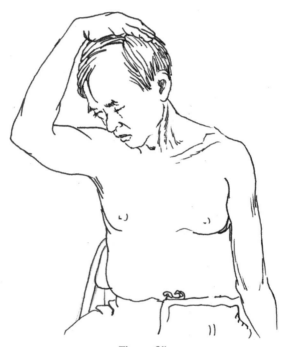

Figure 25

Exercise two: Sternocleidomastoid on one side

This next exercise is intended to provide stretch to one of the major muscles that runs diagonally across the front and side of the neck and has attachments at the collar bone and the back of the skull. Known as the sternocleidomastoid (SCM), this is one of the muscles most frequently involved in ST. The left SCM's normal action is to rotate the head toward the right while also tucking the chin downward to the chest (see Figure 11). The movements in this particular exercise are somewhat complex, and will require some patience and practice to be performed correctly. We will illustrate stretching for the left SCM. The entire procedure may be reversed if you require stretching of the right SCM.

In order to stretch the left SCM, begin in a seated or standing position. Grasp the handhold behind or underneath you with your left hand (Figure 26). Now lean your body slightly so that your left shoulder is pulled downward. If you relax your shoulder, you will find that your collarbone is pulled downward. Now slowly rotate your head toward the left side (the side being stretched). Once your

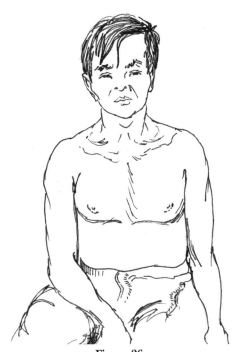

Figure 26

head has been rotated as far as it can comfortably go, begin tilting your head backward so that your chin moves toward the ceiling. Now tilt your head slightly so that your right ear moves closer to your right shoulder (Figure 27). As you do this, you may feel a stretching sensation from your left collarbone to the side of neck. Hold at the point you feel stretch but not pain. After 30 seconds, the feeling of stretch may begin to subside. At this point, you may increase the stretch a little further by cupping the fingers of your left hand around your chin and slowly and gently pushing upwards. As always, stop if you feel pain. Hold this position for 10 more seconds, then slowly release and relax.

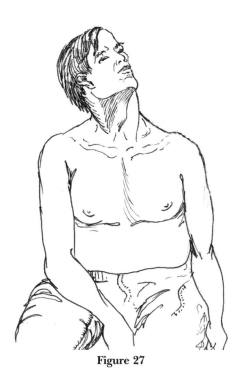

Figure 27

Exercise three: Sternocleidomastoid on both sides

The next exercise is a simple alternative stretch for the SCM that stretches both sides at once, and may be useful for individuals with anterocollis (see Figure 7). This is best done in a seated position in a chair with some support for the back (Figure 28). Simply grasp a handhold behind or underneath you with both hands. Slowly lean your body backward to pull down your shoulders. Allow your shoulder muscles to relax, pulling down your collarbones. Keep your head in the neutral position facing directly ahead. Now, slowly tilt your head backward so that your chin moves toward the ceiling (Figure 29). You should feel a stretching sensation in the front and side of your neck. Do not hunch up your shoulders; allow them to relax and be pulled downward. Hold at the point where you feel stretch but not unusual pain. Hold this position for 30 seconds, then slowly release and relax.

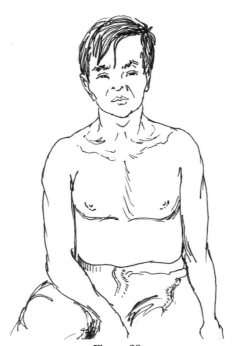

Figure 28

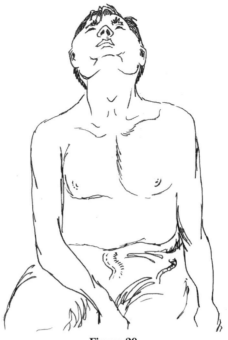

Figure 29

Exercise four: Trapezius, levator scapuli, sternocleidomastoid, and scalenes

The next exercise is intended to provide stretch for the muscles that lift the shoulder upwards and tilt the head directly sideways, mainly the trapezius and levator scapuli, but also the scalenes and sternocleidomastoid. This exercise is useful for persons who have lateral-collis (see Figure 10). We have selected the left-sided muscles for illustration. The entire procedure may be reversed if you require stretching of the right-sided muscles.

Starting from the seated or standing position, grasp a handhold beside you with your left hand (Figure 30). Lean your body to the right while relaxing your shoulder muscles and allowing your shoulder to be pulled downward. Now, tilt your head sideways to the right. You may feel a stretching sensation from the shoulder to the side of the neck. Hold this position for 30 seconds. You may feel the sensation of stretching begin to subside. At this point, you can increase the stretch a little further by placing your right hand over the top of your head and slowly and gently pulling to the right (Figure 31). Stop if you feel any unusual pain. Hold this position for another 10 seconds, then slowly release and relax.

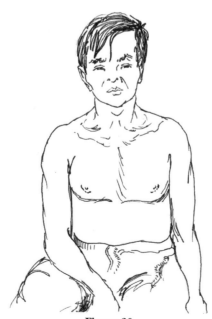

Figure 30

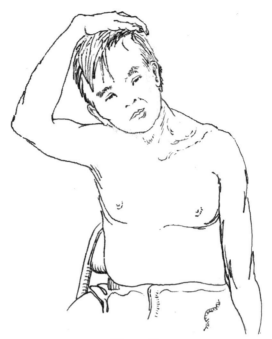

Figure 31

Exercise five: Splenius capitis

The next exercise is intended to provide stretch to several muscles in the back of the neck, mainly the splenius capitis (SC). This muscle starts at the neck bones and runs diagonally upward and outward to the base of the skull. The normal action of the right SC is to pull the head backwards and rotate it slightly to the right side (similar to Figure 18). This exercise is similar to exercise 1, but is more specific for the SC. We will illustrate stretching for the right SC. The entire procedure may be reversed if you require stretching of your left SC.

To stretch the right SC, start in the seated or standing position. First rotate your head toward the left, then tilt your head downward, tucking your chin toward your chest (Figure 32). You may begin feeling a stretching sensation in the back of your neck, on one or both sides. Hold this position for 30 seconds. You may feel the stretching sensation begin to subside. At this point, you may increase the stretch a little further by placing your fingers against the side of your chin and gently pushing to rotate your chin toward your left shoulder (Figure 33). Hold this position for another 10 seconds, then slowly release and relax.

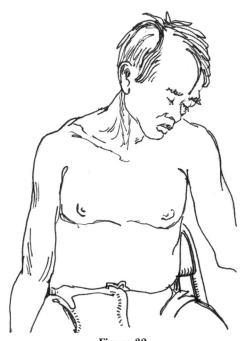

Figure 32

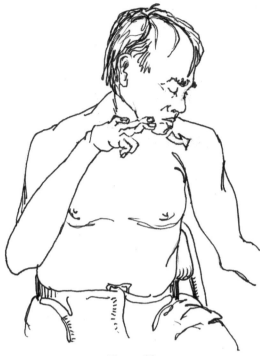

Figure 33

STRENGTHENING EXERCISES

The next set of exercises is designed to strengthen the antagonist muscles. Strengthening these muscles can help to bring your head back to the neutral position. To strengthen any muscle, it is necessary to use it to exert a force against resistance. Thus, to perform these exercises, you will need a suitable object against which to push. A pillow-sized block of soft foam rubber works best and may be obtained from a medical supply store or pharmacy. A larger, thick block of foam is best. Suitable thicker foam pillows may also be found in department and bedding stores. Most of the following exercises can be modified for performance in the sitting, standing, or lying position. In most cases, resistance supplied by an opposing hand or fingers can be substituted for the foam block or pillow, allowing the exercises to be performed in almost any situation. If you are not able to perform an exercise against resistance, try the movement by itself at first, using no type of resistance.

Exercise six: Sternocleidomastoid on one side

This exercise is designed to strengthen the SCM muscle on one side. Overactivity of the *right* sternocleidomastoid produces rotational torticollis toward the *left* (Figure 34), in which case strengthening of the *left* sternocleidomastoid is required. This entire procedure may be reversed if you require strengthening of your right SCM.

To strengthen the left SCM, start in a seated position parallel to a wall. Your right shoulder should just barely touch the wall. Place the foam block on top of your right shoulder flush with the wall (Figure 35). Place the side of your face snugly against the block. Now turn your head slowly as if looking to your right. Rotate your head until you are pressing as hard as you comfortably can (Figure 36). Hold for 30 seconds, then release and relax. Repeat this exercise three to five times per exercise session. Increase as tolerated. Some people may only be able to perform this exercise without a pillow; resistance provided by placing a hand on the side of the face may suffice. Others may not be able to push against a resistance at all.

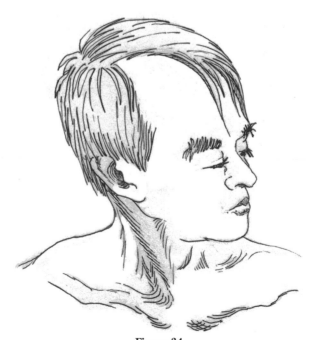

Figure 34

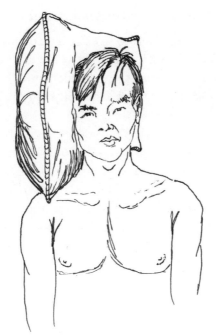

Figure 35

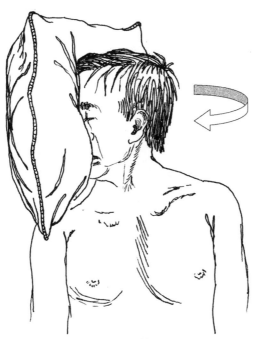

Figure 36

Exercise seven: Trapezius and levator scapuli

The next exercise is intended to strengthen the muscles that elevate the shoulder and shoulder blade, mainly the trapezius and the levator scapuli. We have selected the left-sided muscles for illustration. The entire procedure may be reversed if you require strengthening of the right-sided muscles.

To strengthen the left-sided muscles, start in the seated or standing position. Grasp a handhold beside you with your left hand. Now slowly shrug your left shoulder without moving your head (Figure 37). Remember that the pulling should be done with your shoulder shrug only. Try to keep your arm straight and do not try to lift by bending your arm at the elbow. Pull with your shoulder muscles as hard as you comfortably can, hold for 30 seconds, then slowly release and relax. Repeat this exercise three to five times per exercise session. Increase as tolerated to a maximum of 12 repetitions.

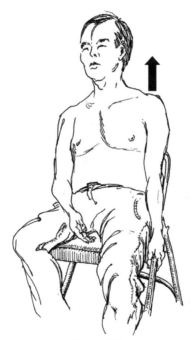

Figure 37

Exercise eight: Splenius capitis and others on one side

This exercise is designed to strengthen the muscles that lie along the back of the neck on either side of the neck bones. These include the diagonally running SC and other deeper muscles. The left SC tilts the head backward and turns the chin slightly toward the left. Movement produced mainly by the left SC is depicted in Figure 21. This person requires strengthening of the right-sided SC (he or she should also strengthen the left SCM). We have selected the right SC for illustration. The entire procedure may be reversed if you require strengthening of your left SC.

To strengthen your right SC, start the exercise lying on your back with the foam pillow underneath your head (Figure 38). Rotate your head approximately 45 degrees to the right. Now tilt your head backwards, pushing into the foam pillow (Figure 39). Try to push against the block with the part of your head immediately behind and above your right ear. Push as hard as you comfortably can, hold for 10 seconds, then slowly release and relax. Repeat this exercise three to five times per exercise session. Increase as tolerated, to a maximum of 12 repetitions.

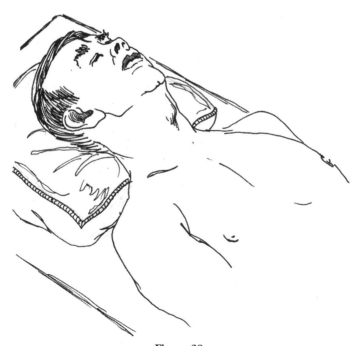

Figure 38

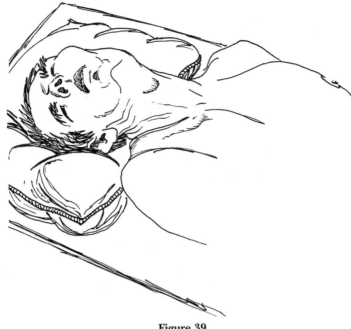

Figure 39

Exercise nine: Sternocleidomastoids on both sides

This is an alternative exercise that can be used if both the right and left SCM muscles need to be strengthened. It may be useful for individuals with retrocollis (see Figure 8). Start by lying flat on your back (Figure 40). Now lift your head straight upwards, tilting your chin slightly toward your chest. If desired, push against your forehead with two fingers as shown to provide resistance (Figure 41). Hold this position for 10 seconds, then slowly release and relax. Repeat this exercise three to five times per exercise session. Increase as tolerated, to a maximum of 12 repetitions.

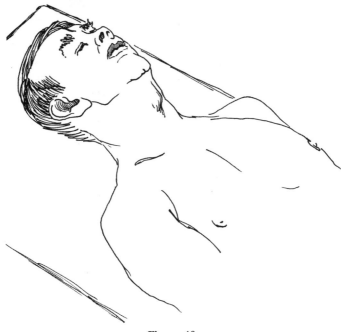

Figure 40

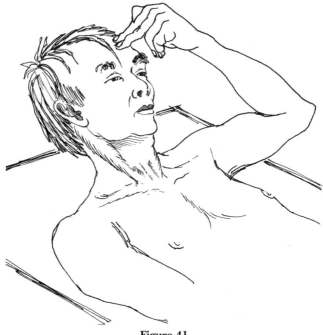

Figure 41

Exercise ten: Sternocleidomastoid, trapezius, levator scapuli, and scalenes

This exercise is designed to strengthen the muscles that tilt the head sideways and elevate the shoulder, including the sternocleidomastoid, trapezius, and levator scapuli. The individual shown in Figure 10 has lateralcollis produced by overactivity of left-sided muscles, and requires strengthening on the right. We have selected the right-sided muscles for illustration. The entire procedure may be reversed if you require strengthening of your left-sided muscles.

To strengthen the right-sided muscles, begin in the seated position on a chair with your right shoulder touching the wall. Place the foam pillow on top of your right shoulder flush with the wall, and place the side of your head snugly against the pillow (Figure 42). Now tilt your head directly sideways to the right, pushing into the foam pillow (Figure 43). Push as hard as you comfortably can, hold for 10 seconds, then slowly release and relax. Repeat this exercise three to five times per exercise session. Increase as tolerated up to 12 repetitions. Some individuals may only be able to perform this

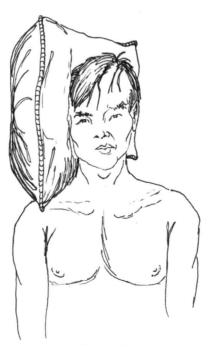

Figure 42

exercise without a pillow; resistance provided by the hand against the side of the face may suffice. Others may only be able to perform the movement against no resistance at all.

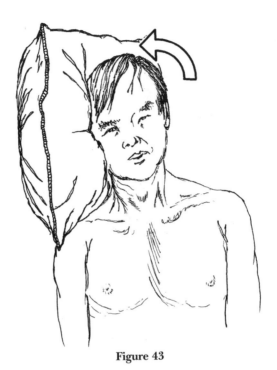

Figure 43

Exercise eleven: Splenius capitis and others on both sides

This next exercise is designed to strengthen all of the muscles that tilt the head straight backwards. These lie along the back of the neck on either side of the spine, including the SC. This exercise may be useful for people with anterocollis, as depicted in Figure 7. Begin by lying on your back on a firm surface with the foam pillow underneath your head (Figure 44). Tilt your head straight backward, pushing into the foam block (Figure 45). Push as hard as you comfortably can, hold for 10 seconds, then slowly release and relax. Repeat this exercise three to five times per exercise session. Increase as tolerated up to 12 repetitions.

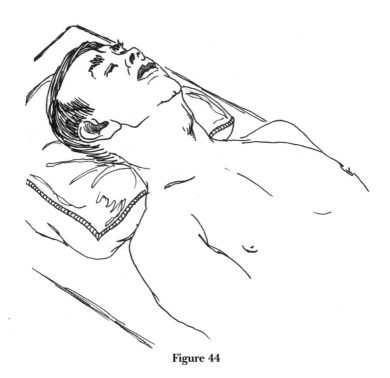

Figure 44

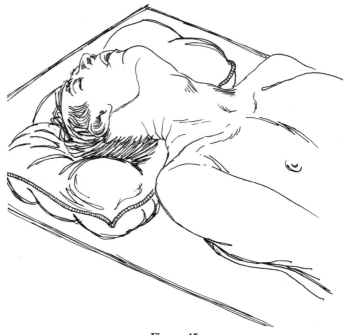

Figure 45

A

Resources

Congratulations! You've just completed the first step in learning to live with ST—educating yourself about the disorder. There are other things you can do that are generally helpful. Joining a support group, such as the National Spasmodic Torticollis Association, can provide encouragement, camaraderie, and information on the latest medical advances and treatments for ST. Having ST is not a hopeless situation, and many times others with the disorder enjoy sharing their coping techniques. Maintaining a sense of good general health through diet and exercise will help as well. It's important to maintain contact with your doctor so that an effective treatment strategy can be developed.

OTHER SOURCES OF INFORMATION

The organizations listed below are rich sources of information on ST and other dystonias. They offer reading materials, books, and videos on these subjects, and they may assist you in finding a local support group or a specialist who treats ST in your area.

The National Spasmodic Torticollis Association
NSTA
9920 Talbert Avenue, Room 233
Fountain Valley, CA 92708
Phone: 714-378-7837
www.torticollis.org

Dystonia Medical Research Foundation
One East Wacker Drive, Suite 2430
Chicago, IL 60601-1905
Phone: 312-755-0198
www.dystonia-foundation.org

We Move (Worldwide Education and Awareness for Movement Disorders)
204 West 84th Street
New York, NY 10024
Phone: 800-437-MOV2
Fax: 212-875-8389
E-mail: wemove@wemove.org
Web site: www.wemove.org

Benign Essential Blepharospasm Research Foundation
P.O. Box 12468
Beaumont, TX 77726-2468
Phone: 409-832-0788
Fax: 409-832-0890
E-mail: bebrf@ih2000.net

The Parkinson's and Movement Disorder Foundation
9940 Talbert Avenue
Fountain Valley, CA 92708
Phone: 714-378-5071
www.pmdf.org

RECOMMENDED BOOKS

Treat Your Own Neck, by Robin McKenzie, published by Orthopaedic Physical Therapy Products, 1997. ISBN 0-47300-209-4.

Spasmodic Torticollis Handbook of Rehabilitative Physiotherapy, Jean-Pierre Bleton, published by Editions Frison-Roche, Paris 1994. ISBN 2-87671-155-9.

VIDEO

Physical Therapy and Exercises for Spasmodic Torticollis, produced by the National Spasmodic Torticollis Association, see contact information above.

B

Glossary

Abductor: Muscles that move two body parts away from each other.

Acetylcholine: A *neurotransmitter* used extensively within the CNS and the parasympathetic nervous system.

Adductors: Muscles that move two body parts closer together.

Advil®: A brand name over-the-counter pain medication; generic name *ibuprofen.*

Agonist: For the purposes of this book, this is the primary muscle or set of muscles that is involuntarily contracting and pulling the head and neck into abnormal posture in *spasmodic torticollis.*

Aleve®: A brand name over-the-counter pain medication; generic name *naproxen.*

Alpha-receptor agonist: A pharmaceutical category of medications that may be used to treat muscle spasms and pain.

Alprazolam: The generic name for *Xanax®.*

Amitriptyline: The generic name for *Elavil®.*

Anoxia: Any state of oxygen deprivation; this may lead to brain damage.

Antagonist: For the purposes of this book, this is any muscle or set of muscles that can oppose the pulling force of *agonists* to move the head and neck back towards normal position.

Anterocollis: Forward tilting of the head, tucking the chin into the chest. This is the most difficult abnormal head posture to treat medically.

Anticholinergic: A pharmaceutical category of medications that may be used to treat movement disorders. These medications inhibit the actions of *acetylcholine* in some locations and thus diminish the effects of the *parasympathetic nervous system.*

Antidepressant: A medication used to treat depression.

Antipsychotic: Synonymous with *neuroleptic*. A psychiatric medication used to treat disorders characterized by hallucinations, delusions, or agitated behavior. Most antipsychotics block the action of the brain chemical dopamine. They may cause movement disorders.

Artane®: An *anticholinergic* medication that may be used to treat movement disorders; generic name *trihexphenidyl*.

Ativan®: A sedative medication of the *benzodiazepine* class that may be used to treat *movement disorders*; generic name *lorazepam*.

Atlanto-axial dislocation: A slippage of the two topmost cervical vertebrae that results in abnormal head posture.

Atrophy: Muscle shrinkage and deterioration. This will occur if the motor nerve that delivers signals to a muscle is cut, chronically compressed, or otherwise disrupted.

Axon: The long wire-like process extending outward from a neuron through which the neuron sends out its electrical and chemical signals.

Baclofen: An antispasicidy medication that enhances the activity of GABA.

Basal ganglia: Several berry-sized clusters of neurons deep within the brain. They are an integral part of the extrapyramidal motor system. They receive and integrate the varied sensory input information and use it to modulate the output of the pyramidal motor system.

Basal ganglia disorders: This term encompasses most *movement disorders*. Most such disorders have their primary site of abnormality in the *basal ganglia*.

Benadryl®: A medication with *anticholinergic* properties that can be used to treat acute *dystonia* or *dyskinesia*; generic name *diphenhydramine*.

Benzodiazepine: A pharmaceutical category of sedative medications that may be used to treat movement disorders.

Benztropine mesylate: The generic name for Cogentin®.

Blepharospasm: A focal dystonia affecting the facial muscles that squeeze the eyelids closed.

Botox®: A brand name of *botulinum toxin* type A.

Botulinum toxin: The nerve toxin produced by the bacterium *Clostridium botulinum*. It is the most commonly used *chemodenervation* medication.

Botulism: A muscle paralyzing disease caused by infection with the bacterium *Clostridium botulinum* through a wound or by ingestion of its toxin in spoiled food.

Bromocriptine: The generic name for *Parlodel®*.

Carbidopa: One of the ingredients of *Sinemet®*. It protects the active ingredient, *levodopa*, from becoming metabolized before it can enter the brain.

Catapress®: A medication in the *alpha-receptor agonist* class that may be used to treat muscle spasms and pain; generic name *clonidine*.

Celexa®: An antidepressant medication in the *SSRI* class than may help relieve pain associated with neurologic conditions; generic name *citalopram*.

Central nervous system: For purposes of this book, this includes the brain and spinal cord.

Cervical dystonia: Synonymous with spasmodic torticollis.

Cervicalgia: Neck pain.

Cervical spine: The portion of the spinal column in the neck.

Cervix: The neck.

Chemodenervation: The injections of a medication into a muscle or nerve to either destroy the nerve or disrupt its connections to the muscle. The targeted muscle then becomes weakened or paralyzed.

Citalopram: The generic name for *Celexa®*.

Clonazepam: The generic name for *Klonopin®*.

Clonidine: The generic name for *Catapress®*.

Chlordiazepoxide: The generic name for *Librium®*.

Clostridium botulinum: The species of bacteria that produces *botulinum toxin*.

CNS: Central nervous system. For purposes of this book, this includes the brain and spinal cord.

Cogentin®: An *anticholinergic* medication used to treat *movement disorders*. The generic name is *benztropine mesylate*.

Compazine®: A medication that blocks the action of *dopamine*. It can cause transient acute *dystonia* or *dyskinesia*. Rarely, it can lead to a permanent movement disorder. The generic name is *prochlorperazine*.

Computed tomography: A computer-assisted X-ray imaging technique.

CT: Computed tomography.

Dantrium: The generic name for *Dantrolene®*.

Dantrolene®: An antispasticity medication that works inside muscle tissue. The generic name is *dantrium*.

Deep brain stimulation: The surgical implantation of a battery-driven device that disrupts the electrical signals of the *basal ganglia* and *extrapyramidal motor system* by means of electrode wires that are inserted into the brain. It is used mainly to treat the symptoms of severe *Parkinson's disease.*

Diazepam: The generic name for *Valium®.*

Diphenhydramine: The generic name for *Benadryl®.*

Dopamine: One of the principal *neurotransmitters* of the *basal ganglia* and *extrapyramidal motor system.* Drugs or medical conditions that disrupt the activity of dopamine may cause movement disorders. Some drugs that modify dopamine activity may be used to treat movement disorders.

Dopamine agonist: A pharmaceutical class of medications that mimic the action of *dopamine* in the brain. These are most often used to treat *Parkinson's disease.*

Dopamine-responsive dystonia: A small percentage of movement disorders (other than *Parkinson's disease*) that improve with the administration of *Sinemet®* or *dopamine agonists.*

Dyskinesia: Involuntary movement of one or more body parts. It often coexists with dystonia in the same body part. It is a frequent manifestation of movement disorders.

Dysport®: A brand name of *botulinum toxin* type A, marketed in Europe and used in the United States in experimental studies.

Dystonia: Sustained involuntary increased muscle tone in one or more body parts. This often results in abnormal posture of the affected part. It is a frequent manifestation of movement disorders.

Elavil®: A *tricyclic antidepressant* that has some *anticholinergic* properties. It can be used to treat the pain associated with neurologic disorders and may mildly diminish *dystonia.* The generic name is *amitriptyline.*

Electromyography: A diagnostic technique used to monitor and record the electrical activity in contracting muscles. It can also be used to guide the placement of *chemodenervation* injections.

EMG: *Electromyography.*

Encephalitis: Any infection or inflammation affecting the brain.

Epilepsy: A neurologic disorder of the brain resulting in seizures. This is not a movement disorder, but seizures can manifest as convulsive movements with or without impairment or loss of consciousness.

Extrapyramidal disorders: This term encompasses most *movement disorders*. The primary site of abnormality is usually in the *basal ganglia*.

Extrapyramidal motor system: A subsystem of the motor system in the CNS. The extrapyramidal system controls and modulates the output of the pyramidal system, acting as a "fine tuner" of movements and preventing excessive movements. The basal ganglia are an integral part of the extrapyramidal system.

Fibromyalgia: A medical condition characterized by pain in muscles and other soft tissues.

Fluoxetine: The generic name for *Prozac*®.

Foramina: "Windows." These are gaps between each of the *vertebrae* through which nerve roots containing motor and sensory components pass. The foramina are common sites at which such nerves may become compressed or "pinched."

GABA: Gamma-amino butyric acid. A *neurotransmitter* in the brain and spinal cord that has mainly inhibitory properties.

Geste antagoniste: "Sensory trick." This usually consists of brushing one's fingers or hand against the face and neck, and it may help to bring the head position in spasmodic torticollis back to normal.

Halcion®: A sedative medication in the *benzodiazepine* class. The generic name is *triazolam*.

Hemifacial spasm: A focal *dystonia* that affects facial muscles, usually on one side.

Honeymoon period: A brief period of time, usually after awakening, during which symptoms of spasmodic torticollis are diminished.

Hydrocodone: A narcotic drug that is an ingredient in *Vicodin*® and other pain medications.

Ibuprofen: The generic name for Advil®, Motrin®, and other brand name pain medications.

Idiopathic: A descriptive term for any medical condition that seems to arise of its own accord, with no discernible inciting cause.

Imipramine: The generic name for *Tofranil®*.

Klonopin®: A sedative medication in the *benzodiazepine* class that may be used to treat *movement disorders*. The generic name is *clonazepam*.

Laterocollis: Sideways tilting of the head, moving one ear closer to the shoulder on the same side.

Levator scapuli: Neck muscle whose main action is to lift the shoulder blade upward and elevate the shoulder.

Levodopa: An active ingredient in *Sinemet®* and other medications for *Parkinson's disease*. It supplies *dopamine* to the brain.

Librium®: A sedative medication in the *benzodiazepine* class that may be used to treat *movement disorders*.

Lidocaine: An anesthetic agent that can be injected into tissues for local pain relief.

Lorazepam: The generic name for *Ativan®*.

Magnetic resonance spectroscopy: A computerized medical imaging technique using a magnetic field and radio waves.

Meige syndrome: A focal *dyskinesia* affecting muscles of the face.

Metoclopramide: The generic name for *Reglan®*.

Mirapex®: A *dopamine agonist*, a medication that mimics the action of *dopamine*. It is usually used to treat Parkinson's disease. The generic name is *pramipexole*.

Motor nerves: Nerves that branch off from the spinal cord, emerge from the spinal column through *foramina* between each of the *vertebrae*, and carry signals for contraction and movement out to the muscles.

Motor system: Those parts of the brain and spinal cord concerned with moving the muscles and controlling those movements. This can also include motor nerves carrying signals to the muscles.

Motrin®: A brand name over-the-counter pain medication.

Movement disorder: Any neurologic disorder characterized by abnormal posture or movement in one or more body parts.

MRI: Magnetic resonance imaging.

Myobloc™: A brand name for *botulinum toxin* type B.

Myotomy: A surgical technique in which specific muscles are cut or removed in order to relieve *dystonia.*

Naproxen sodium: The generic name for Aleve® and other brand name pain medications.

Nerve root: Nerve structures that are attached to the spinal cord and pass through the *foramina* between each of the *vertebrae.* They contain sensory components bringing input information to the *CNS,* and motor components sending signals for movement out to the muscles.

Neuroleptic: Synonymous with antipsychotic. A psychiatric medication used to treat disorders characterized by hallucinations, delusions, or agitated behavior. Most neuroleptics block the action of the brain chemical dopamine. They may cause movement disorders.

Neuron: A nerve cell that sends and receives signals. These cells are located in the gray matter of the brain, in the basal ganglia, and in the spinal cord.

Neurotransmitter: A chemical that carries a signal from the terminal end of an axon across a small gap to another *neuron* or muscle cell.

Nortriptyline: The generic name for *Pamelor®.*

Occupational dystonia: A focal *dystonia* affecting any body part that manifests when performing a particular task.

Ocular dystonia: A focal *dystonia* affecting muscles that move the eyeballs.

Orbicularis oculi: The facial muscle that squeezes the eyelids closed.

Oromandibular dystonia: A focal *dystonia* affecting muscles of the mouth and jaws.

Pamelor®: A *tricyclic antidepressant.* It may be used to treat neurologic causes of pain. The generic name is *nortriptyline.*

Paraplegia: Weakness or paralysis of the two lower limbs due to an injury or other disruption of the spinal cord.

Parasympathetic nervous system: A system of *neurons* and nerves that controls many automatic functions of the body. It uses *acetylcholine* as a *neurotransmitter.*

Paresis: Weakness of one or more body parts due to an injury or disruption of any part of the *motor system.*

Parkinson's disease: A movement disorder characterized by tremor of the hands or feet when at rest, increased *resting tone* of muscles resulting in rigidity of the trunk and limbs, a stooped posture, and impairment of balance and gait.

Parlodel®: A *dopamine* agonist, a medication that mimics the action of *dopamine.* It is usually used to treat Parkinson's disease. The generic name is *bromocriptine.*

Paroxetine: The generic name for *Paxil®.*

Paxil®: An antidepressant medication in the *SSRI* class. It may help to relieve pain associated with neurologic conditions. The generic name is *paroxetine.*

Pergolide: The generic name for *Permax®.*

Peripheral nervous system: This includes motor nerves coming out of the spinal cord, the muscles, and sensory nerves carrying information back to the CNS.

Permax®: A *dopamine* agonist, a medication that mimics the action of *dopamine.* It is usually used to treat Parkinson's disease. The generic name is *pergolide.*

Phenol: A solvent that may be used as a *chemodenervation* agent.

Pramipexole: The generic name for *Mirapex®.*

Prochlorperazine: The generic name for *Compazine®.*

Prozac®: An antidepressant medication in the *SSRI* class. It may help relieve pain associated with neurologic conditions. The generic name is *fluoxetine.*

Pyramidal motor system: A subsystem of the motor system in the CNS. The pyramidal system generates and sends out the primary signal for a group of muscles to contract and cause movement.

Radicular: Anything having to do with the motor and sensory *nerve roots* that pass through the *foramina.* Radicular pain is often felt to radiate along the territory of the sensory component of a *nerve root.* Radicular weakness and *atrophy* can occur among muscles supplied by the motor component of a *nerve root.*

Radiculopathy: Any medical condition that affects a nerve root. Radicular pain is often felt to radiate along the territory of the sensory component of a *nerve root.* Radicular weakness and *atrophy* can occur among muscles supplied by the motor component of a *nerve root.*

Rebound effect: A transient worsening of a medical condition or symptom that may occur if a medication being taken to treat it is abruptly discontinued.

Reglan®: A medicine that blocks the action of *dopamine.* It can cause transient acute *dystonia* or *dyskinesia.* Rarely, it can lead to a permanent *movement disorder.* The generic name is *metoclopramide.*

Requip®: A *dopamine* agonist, a medication that mimics the action of *dopamine.* It is usually used to treat Parkinson's disease. The generic name is *ropinirole.*

Resting tone: The low level of electrical excitation and contraction in which all muscles are maintained during wakefulness. Movement disorders are characterized by abnormalities of resting tone.

Restoril®: A sedative medication in the *benzodiazepine* class. The generic name is temazepam.

Retrocollis: Backward tilting of the head, moving the chin upward, away from the chest.

Rheumatic heart disease: An inflammation of heart tissue associated with a certain bacterial infection. *Sydenham's chorea* is one of the long-term sequelae of this condition.

Rhizotomy: A surgical technique in which spinal nerve roots are cut in order to relieve pain or muscular *dystonia.*

Ropinirole: The generic name for *Requip®.*

Scalenes: Neck muscles whose main action is to pull the neck to the side and tilt the head toward the same side.

Selective peripheral denervation: A surgical technique in which the *motor nerve* branches to specific muscles are cut in order to relieve *dystonia.*

SSRI: *Selective serotonin reuptake inhibitor.*

Selective serotonin reuptake inhibitors: A subclass of *antidepressant* medications.

Semispinalis capitis: Neck muscle whose main action is to bend the head and neck backward.

Sensory nerves: Nerves that carry sensory input information from the skin, joints, and muscles to the CNS. They enter the spinal column through the *foramina* between each of the *vertebrae,* merge with the spinal cord, then relay their signals to sensory pathways that reach the brain.

Sensory trick: Same as *geste antagoniste.*

Sertraline: The generic name for *Zoloft®.*

Sinemet®: A medication that includes the chemicals *carbidopa* and *levodopa*. Its active ingredient is levodopa, which enters the brain and is turned into *dopamine*. It is most often used to treat *Parkinson's disease*.

SLE: *Systemic lupus erythmatosus.*

Spasmodic dysphonia: A focal *dystonia* affecting the vocal cords that impairs the voice.

Spasmodic torticollis: A neurologic movement disorder characterized by abnormal position or tremor of the head and neck. Also known as *cervical dystonia*.

Splenius capitis: Neck muscle whose main action is to bend the head backward and rotate it slightly to the same side.

Splenius cervicis: Neck muscle whose main action is to bend the neck backward.

Sternocleidomastoid: A neck muscle whose main action is to rotate the head toward the opposite side.

Strabismus: A medical condition in which the eyes are misaligned with each other.

Striatum: Certain parts of the basal ganglia that together receive signals via the neurotransmitter *dopamine;* they are important in the control of movement.

Stroke: A neurologic condition caused by a blockage of a brain artery or by bleeding into the brain. The manifestations of a stroke depend on its size and its location in the brain. Occasionally, it can result in a *movement disorder*.

Sydenham's chorea: A movement disorder characterized by writhing movements of the limbs. It is a long-term sequela of *rheumatic heart disease*.

Systemic lupus erythematosus: A medical disorder of the body's immune system. The manifestations of this disease are multifold; it can produce *movement disorders* if it affects the brain.

Tardive dyskinesia: A late-onset *movement disorder* that arises months or years after the chronic use of medications that interfere with the action of the brain chemical *dopamine*. It is characterized by increased muscle tone and abnormal movements (such as tremor or writhing) in the affected body parts.

Tardive dystonia: A late-onset *movement disorder* that arises months or years after chronic use of medications that interfere with the action of the brain chemical *dopamine*. It is characterized by increased muscle tone and abnormal posture in the affected body parts, and is usually permanent.

Temazepam: The generic name for *Restoril®*.

TENS: *Transepidural nerve stimulator.*

Tension cervicalgia: A temporary disorder characterized by muscle spasms in the neck, aching pain, and a feeling of stiffness. People often hold their head in an abnormal position to avoid pain. This is not a movement disorder.

Thalamotomy: A surgical technique in which a small part of the *basal ganglia* is destroyed. It is used to relieve symptoms of severe *Parkinson's disease.*

Tizanidine: The generic name for *Zanaflex®*.

Tofranil®: A *tricyclic antidepressant*. It may be used to treat neurological causes of pain.

Torticollis: "Twisted neck." An involuntary abnormal posture of the head and neck from any medical condition. This can include developmental or orthopaedic conditions. This term is also used to indicate right or left rotation of the head on its axis.

Transepidural nerve stimulator: An electrical stimulation device attached to the skin and used for pain relief.

Trapezius: A neck muscle whose main action is to lift the shoulder upwards.

Trauma: Physical injury to any body part from an external source.

Triazolam: The generic name for *Halcion®*.

Tricyclic antidepressant: A subclass of *antidepressants.*

Trihexphenidyl: The generic name for *Artane®*.

Valium®: A sedative medication in the *benzodiazepine* class that may be used to treat *movement disorders.*

Vertebra: One of the bones stacked upon one another that form the spinal column.

Vertebrae: Plural of vertebra.

Vicodin®: A brand name pain medication containing a combination of the narcotic hydrocodone and acetaminophen.

Whiplash: A term used to describe the type of neck injury that occurs with a sudden acceleration and deceleration of the body, causing the head and neck to flex back and forth rapidly. This may occur in a motor vehicle collision.

Wilson's disease: A metabolic disorder in which the normal metabolism of the trace mineral copper is disrupted. One of its manifestations is as a movement disorder.

Writer's cramp: A focal *dystonia* affecting arm and hand muscles that manifests during writing or similar tasks.

Wry-neck: In this book, this term is synonymous with *tension cervicalgia*.

Xanax®: A sedative medication in the benzodiazepine class that may be used to treat *movement disorders*.

Zanaflex®: A medication in the *alpha-receptor agonist* class that may be used to treat muscle spasms and pain. The generic name is *tizanidine*.

Zoloft®: An *antidepressant* medication in the *SSRI* class. It may help relieve pain associated with neurological conditions. The generic name is *sertraline*.

Index

Note: Boldface numbers indicate illustrations.

brain surgery, 69–70
bromocriptine (Parlodel), 56
bupivicaine, 59

caffeine, 75
Catapress (*See* clonidine)
causes of spasmodic torticollis,
    33–39
Celexa (*See* citalopram)
central nervous system (CNS), 2
central spinal canal, 66
cervical collars, 74–75
cervical dystonia, v, 1, 3
cervical spinal cord and spine,
    20–21, **20, 67**
chemodenervation, 32, 59, 61–62,
    71
chemotheraphy side effects, 35
chiropractic, 74
chloridiazepoxide (Librium), 53
chorea, 37
citalopram (Celexa), 57
clonazepam (Klonopin), 53
clonidine (Catapress), 55
Clostridium botulinum (*See also*
    botulinum toxin), 61–62
Cogentin (*See* benztropine mesy-
    late)
collars, cervical, 74–75
Compazine (*See* prochlorperazine)
computed tomography (CT), 41,
    44
coping with spasmodic torticollis,
    9–14
copper metabolism disorders,
    37
cramps, 31

dantrolene (Dantrium), 55
deep brain stimulation, 69, 70
defining spasmodic torticollis, v–vi,
    1–8, 1
dependence on drugs, 54
diagnosing spasmodic torticollis,
    9–14, 41–50

diazepam (Valium), 53, 54, 58
diet, 75
diffuse dystonias/dyskinesias, 46
diphenhydramine (Benadryl), 35
discs between vertebrae, 31–32
disfiguration, 11–12
dislocations of cervical spine, 45
dopamine, 19, 34, 35, 37, 55–56
dopamine agonists, 55–56
dopamine–enhancing medications,
    55–57
dopamine–responsive dystonia,
    56
drowning as cause of spasmodic
    torticollis, 36, 43
drug–induced spasmodic
    torticollis, 34, 37, 42–44
dyskinesia, 3, 35, 46
Dysport (*See also* botulinum toxin),
    62, 63
dystonia, 3, 35
Dystonia Medical Research
    Foundation, 97

Elavil (*See* amitryptiline)
electromyography (EMG), 63
encephalitis as cause of spasmodic
    torticollis, 36
excitation of muscles, 15
exercise, 5, 73, 75–100
    strengthening, 89–100
    stretching type, 78–88
extension of muscles, 21, 30
extrapyramidal disorders, 19
extrapyramidal motor system,
    17–18, 37
eyes and dystonias, 48–49

facial dystonias, 48–49
fatigue, 5
fibromyalgia, 55
flexion of muscles, 21, 30
fluoxetine (Prozac), 35
focal limb dystonias, 46–47
foramina, 66